'An invaluable resource for all practitioners
and emotional development of children a
of issues and accompanying activities are presented in an informative and
clear structure with guidance on potential safeguarding and child protection
issues to help ensure "safe" practice. An absolute must for all those who deal
with "challenging" behaviour in our mainstream schools; the book you have
all been waiting for!'

— Alison Chown, Play Therapist, Supervisor and Educational Trainer

'As a teacher of Technology, having such an accessible and easy to use
resource, packed with information that helps with recognising the warning
signs of emotional distress and how this can present in a child's behaviour, is
fantastic. With super ideas for drama-based games and activities that provide
creative and fun ways to overcome these challenges, and with the additional
benefit of providing guidance on when and how to engage other professional
help when necessary, it's a must read.'

— Tom Vaughan, Teacher of Design and Technology, South West England

'A remarkable resource which guides teachers and staff to skilfully utilize
drama, a valuable but often overlooked means of supporting troubled children
in the classroom. The author, a professional drama therapist, deftly combines
theory and practice by identifying familiar behavioural issues, providing
insight regarding the issues and clearly describing innovative techniques and
drama activities to foster emotional growth and healing. Helpfully, a number
of the activities are useable or adaptable for younger children. Whether
coping with a stressful classroom problem or waiting for delayed special
services, this much needed book is a life line for all.'

— Dr. Carol Woodard, Professor Emeritus, State University
College at Buffalo, New York and author of Make-Believe
Play and Story-Based Drama in Early Childhood

'Deeply impressive, moving and accessible. This book takes the reader on an
insightful journey into the world of the troubled child whilst demystifying
creative drama, leaving you empowered with a tool kit of practical, structured
drama techniques that can be embedded into the heart of any nurturing
classroom.'

— Debbie Shotter, Senior Educational Psychologist, Associate
Fellow of the British Psychological Society

CREATIVE DRAMA
FOR EMOTIONAL SUPPORT

by the same author

Dramatherapy and Family Therapy in Education
Essential Pieces of the Multi-Agency Jigsaw
Penny McFarlane and Jenny Harvey
Foreword by Sue Jennings
ISBN 978 1 84905 216 0
eISBN 978 0 85700 451 2

of related interest

Creative Coping Skills for Children
Emotional Support through Arts and Crafts Activities
Bonnie Thomas
ISBN 978 1 84310 921 1
eISBN 978 1 84642 954 5

Make-Believe Play and Story-Based Drama in Early Childhood
Let's Pretend!
Carol Woodard with Carri Milch
ISBN 978 1 84905 899 5
eISBN 978 0 85700 639 4

Helping Children to Cope with Change, Stress and Anxiety
A Photocopiable Activities Book
Deborah M. Plummer
Illustrated by Alice Harper
ISBN 978 1 84310 960 0
eISBN 978 0 85700 366 9

The Big Book of Therapeutic Activity Ideas for Children and Teens
Inspiring Arts-Based Activities and Character Education Curricula
Lindsey Joiner
ISBN 978 1 84905 865 0
eISBN 978 0 85700 447 5

Creating Children's Art Games for Emotional Support
Vicky Barber
ISBN 978 1 84905 163 7
eISBN 978 0 85700 409 3

CREATIVE DRAMA
FOR EMOTIONAL SUPPORT

Activities and Exercises for Use in the Classroom

Penny McFarlane

Foreword by Sylvia Wheadon

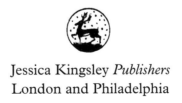

Jessica Kingsley *Publishers*
London and Philadelphia

Figures 1–25 are reprinted with permission from Stuart McFarlane and MacKenzie Slater-Beggs. Permissions for all case studies were kindly granted by the families of the young people featured.

First published in 2012
by Jessica Kingsley Publishers
116 Pentonville Road
London N1 9JB, UK
and
400 Market Street, Suite 400
Philadelphia, PA 19106, USA

www.jkp.com

Library of Congress Cataloging in Publication Data
McFarlane, Penny.
Creative drama for emotional support : activities and exercises for use in the classroom / Penny McFarlane ; foreword by Sylvia Wheadon.
p. cm.
Includes bibliographical references and index.
ISBN 978-1-84905-251-1 (alk. paper)
1. Drama--Therapeutic use. 2. School children. I. Title.
RC489.P7M395 2012
616.89'1653--dc23
2012005379

British Library Cataloguing in Publication Data
A CIP catalogue record for this book is available from the British Library

ISBN 978 1 84905 251 1
eISBN 978 0 85700 529 8

Printed and bound in Great Britain

To my father, for many reasons

CONTENTS

Foreword 11

ACKNOWLEDGEMENTS. 13

DISCLAIMER AND NOTES OF CAUTION 15

PREFACE: WHY DRAMA? 17

    Value and meaning of play 17
    How to use this book 18
    What this book covers. 20
    What this book does *not* cover 22

Introduction. 23
    What are the issues?. 23
    How can we recognize the issues? 24
    What can we do about the issues?. 28

Activities 39
    What to do at the beginning of a session 39
    Issues, Behaviours and Supporting Activities. 42

    Abuse. 42

    Anger. 48

    Anxiety 54

    Attachment 58

    Bereavement. 66

    Bullying. 75

    Change or transition 83

Compulsive lying 87

Depression. 91

Lack of self-esteem/confidence. 96

Learnt behaviour 103

Neglect 106

Nightmares. 111

Parental separation. 115

Sibling rivalry 122

Socially inappropriate behaviour. 129

Speech problems 134

Trauma and shock 139

Conclusion 143

What to do at the end of a session 143

Appendix 1: Group Bonding Games 149

Appendix 2: Index of Issues and Supporting Activities. 151

Appendix 3: References, Useful Resources and Further Reading. 153

Index 155

FOREWORD

The author Penny McFarlane has previously published a book entitled *Dramatherapy: Developing Emotional Stability*; she has a Master's Degree in professional writing as well as many years of experience in schools as a qualified teacher and dramatherapist with children who need emotional support.

It is these experiences that have led Penny to recognize that, more than anything, teaching staff, teaching assistants and support workers need information to help them understand behaviours that manifest into disturbances in the classroom or playground.

This book converts the unique quality of her experiences into a highly practical, easy to comprehend choice of activities and exercises, which can be safely used in the classroom by those trained to look after children, but who have no previous therapeutic experience, or training.

The activities and exercises are explained in clear and simple language, as well as when, how and why the use of these exercises may be beneficial.

Penny also devotes sections of the book to explain that if it is apparent that a child needs extra help, when to refer on for specialist intervention.

The book would also be a valuable practical tool for any trained therapist.

Sylvia Wheadon
Educational Trainer, Dramatherapist,
Psychotherapist, Psychodramatist

ACKNOWLEDGEMENTS

I would like to thank all those who have supported me in the writing of this book, in particular Sylvia, Jenny, Annie and Nina, who have taken the time to read, advise, enthuse and quibble. Their respective, professional expertise and knowledge has given me the confidence to offer the information contained here in the hope that it will empower those who are already caring for troubled children.

In particular I would like to acknowledge Sylvia Wheadon for her continuing enthusiasm for, and interest in, my work, and Mackenzie Slater-Beggs for his lovely ideas for the illustrations.

As always I am grateful for the continuing love and support of my family: my daughters Leonie and Alexine and my husband Stuart who has slaved long and hard in his new career as an illustrator!

ACKNOWLEDGMENTS

DISCLAIMER
AND NOTES OF CAUTION

The misapplication of dramatherapy methods by an untrained person could result in extreme client distress. Dramatherapists are professionally trained at postgraduate level and are subject to a Code of Practice and Ethics as laid down by their own professional body. The author accepts no liability for any such malpractice and advises that the *Notes of caution* as laid down in this book are adhered to *at all times*.

PREFACE
Why Drama?

VALUE AND MEANING OF PLAY

'You can't sit there grandma! Bisa Bisa is sitting there!', my four-year-old tells her horrified grandmother just as she is about to manoeuvre herself into the small space left between the piles of shopping on the back seat of the car. The expression on my daughter's face is so outraged that for a moment grandma thinks she actually *has* sat on a small child.

In her book on playtherapy, Saralea Chazan tells us that 'Play occupies a realm outside of everyday events. It has to do with imaginings and trial action. Anything is possible, and no consequences need intrude' (Chazan 2002, p.19). It is through this world of make believe that a child learns to experiment with the 'what if?' What if there was another little girl in the back of the car? What if grandma did sit on her? By gently moving aside some cat food, grandma enters the game of make believe and receives a winning smile for her pains. My daughter knows that her grandma knows that Bisa Bisa isn't really there, but it doesn't matter. The scenario is a stage on which the actors can play with, and stretch, the boundaries of reality. How else can a child learn to explore the intricate and infinite complexities of life? How else can she reduce her world to a size that is both manageable and safe?

It is through their play that children communicate their fears, hopes and desires to us. Older children may be able to tell us that their mother is so depressed she is unable to look after them but a younger child will only play with a big dragon puppet who is gobbling up the mummy tiger and preventing the baby tiger from reaching her.

Sue Jennings, author of many books on play and dramatherapy, questions whether play actually starts in utero in the interaction between the mother and her unborn child. The mother will talk to her growing baby and answer herself *as the child* (Jennings 1999).

Certainly this phenomenon is apparent in a healthy attachment between mother and child once the child is born, while its absence may be a contributing factor in insecure attachment patterns (see 'Attachment', pp.58–65).

It is through the 'doing' rather than the 'watching' that we learn. Depending on their learning style some people (this is my excuse anyway!) find it impossible to remember such things as directions or how to mend a fuse unless they have actually driven there or mended one themselves! With so many things to learn about the world, it is crucial to their development that children be encouraged to use the medium of dramatic play to explore not only the boundaries of what *is*, but also the possibilities of what *might be*.

Through creative drama activities a child is able to comprehend what is and what might be, not only in his mind, but also by feeling it in his body. Being told you have the ability to do amazing things is not as empowering as actually *doing* them, if only in role-play. Fighting off dragons with a shield you have made yourself, pulling a sword from a stone with your classmates as witnesses, or flying around the room as Superman or another of your favourite heroes is something you will remember far longer than just writing or talking about it. Moreover, and more importantly, it is something you will remember in your heart, rather than only in your head.

HOW TO USE THIS BOOK
Who is this book for?

This book has been written as a response to direct enquiries and indirect mumblings about what can be done to help the myriad children in our schools who either have emotional problems which are deemed too low level to be dealt with by the relevant professional bodies, or who are on a long waiting list for assessment and support. This book is for all staff who have to deal with such children in the meantime and feel out of their depth or stuck for ideas. From experience I know that there are many caring and capable adults out there who, finding themselves overwhelmed by the issues and problems these children face, wish, from the bottom of their hearts, they could understand them better and have more resources to help.

It is, however, most definitely not my intention to produce material that tries to turn a layperson into a would-be therapist. Throughout the Activities the 'Notes of caution' deal specifically with the cut-off point at which professional therapeutic support is not only desirable but also mandatory, the point beyond which it would be dangerous to proceed. The exercises in this book should be used only to *support* children with emotional problems, and not in any way to *treat* them.

Having said this, I must own that, coming from a background of dramatherapy and having seen the benefits of being able to work therapeutically with children, it would also be my hope that this book might inspire others to understand their limitations and want to train to become therapists in their own right.

What do you need to be able to use this book?

Although this book has been specifically designed to be appropriate for those with little or no therapeutic training, it is *expressly advised* that it is not suitable for those who are completely new to working with children. At least a year's experience in this field together with some special needs/counselling/listening training would be a minimum requirement to be able to use the activities safely and effectively. In all cases it is advised that anyone feeling out of their depth should refer to a professional or undertake the necessary training. For example, no one would feel comfortable trying to work with a family without having had some sort of training in family matters (see 'Bereavement', pp.66–74). Some schools already have their own internal support network, for example, a special educational needs (SEN) teacher or specially appointed pastoral staff, and any member of staff with concerns over a child should obviously always take advantage of this assistance before looking elsewhere.

A safe, uninterrupted space (if such a thing exists in a school environment!) allows the activities to be more effective, especially in one-to-one work. Since trust is a prerequisite to any emotionally supportive work, it is helpful if a child can be sure that strangers are not going to barge into his space at any given moment. Even in group work it is important to segregate this sort of input from the normal routine of the school day, not only to enable it to be more convincing but also to emphasize its importance.

Resources and materials

All the activities require few or no resources. A general kit bag would be as follows: coloured pens or pencils of some sort, paper and card, a roll of wallpaper (for use on the reverse side), lengths (at least a metre square) of coloured material and various chairs and cushions. Dressing-up clothes make the acting more fun but are not obligatory since, with a little imagination, it is surprising what can be done with the lengths of material.

WHAT THIS BOOK COVERS

The main component of the book is the Activities section. For ease of reading and application this section has been divided into 18 main issues that may affect children of school age today. This section begins with suggestions for games and activities that may be useful as warm-up exercises. Within each activity there is a description of the specific issue, which has, of necessity, been curtailed to the background information most relevant and useful (in my opinion) to any layperson having to deal with children's emotional problems.

The next section within the activity is a description of some behaviours most likely to emerge from this issue with information on specific age-related behaviours, if relevant. Again, if appropriate, general supporting activities with desired outcomes are offered together with any areas for concern and suggestions for when a child should be referred on to other professional agencies. Additionally, questions to ask oneself when dealing with specific behaviour are included in some of the sections.

In order to distinguish between the drama and other activities, the drama activities themselves are referred to as exercises and are explained in an easy step-by-step style with a list of resources required and suggestions for application, for example, suitability for individual or group work, etc. Reasons are given as to why this particular exercise has been chosen as well as what it is trying to achieve. Further explanations on this are given in the Introduction, in 'Underpinnings of dramatherapy', pp.32–34. If appropriate, alternative age-related exercises are also offered within each activity.

Some exercises include extension activities such as discussion, drawing or craftwork, while suggestions for additional activities applicable to this issue may be found in the 'Further activities' section. Finally, suggestions as to how these particular activities and exercises may support other issues are given under 'Other issues addressed'. The line drawings that accompany some of the exercises have been included as a memory aid.

Occasionally it has been necessary to introduce a 'Note of caution' into the exercises to enable the member of staff concerned to understand where support leaves off and therapy takes over. *It is strongly advised that these recommendations are adhered to.*

The Introduction to the book takes a brief look in a more general way at the issues facing our children in schools today and refers to some research findings from an inner-city arts therapies project. Presenting behaviours in both the classroom and playground are discussed and some suggestions made for the way in which they may be recognized and initially supported.

General and differentiated approaches are then considered before a more in-depth explanation of the underpinnings of one particular model of dramatherapy is offered as a way of giving the background to the reasons for the choice of the activities and drama exercises. *This particular section is offered as background information only and it is not intended that it be used as a training manual.*

The reason for the inclusion of this particular section is not only to support the layperson in an understanding of how a child's external circumstances can affect his emotional development, but also to act as an introduction to the world of metaphor and symbol through which a small child communicates as well as giving some examples of the different ways the child might view the world.

Finally, in the Introduction there is a section on 'Using drama techniques' in which some of the exercises and more technical terms such as 'sculpting', 'mirroring' and 'freeze frames' are explained in more detail (see pp.35–37).

The Conclusion considers what to do at the end of a session, which activities might be suitable for the acknowledgement of a group and how to ensure a child returns to his class in a calm and controlled state.

As well as the References section, the Appendices include ideas for group bonding activities, a cross-reference index comprising a list of issues and suitable activities and a useful resources page and further reading.

In the book, to avoid confusion, the child is referred to as 'he' and the supporting adult as 'she'.

WHAT THIS BOOK DOES *NOT* COVER

This book does not attempt to give an in-depth résumé of safeguarding issues or precise circumstances under which a child should be referred either to social services or other outside agencies. Where there are any concerns whatsoever, the protocol relating to disclosure and child protection, applicable to that particular school or organization, should be followed.

Moreover, this book does not aim to equip the layperson with the tools necessary to make a diagnosis and attempt to act on it in isolation, the objective instead being merely to raise awareness of the issues and resulting behaviours. At all times it is recommended that staff restrict themselves to referring to their line manager and record in as much detail as possible any concerns they may have, always differentiating between what is *factual evidence* and what is either their professional opinion or gut instinct. In this way concerns may be stockpiled and become pieces of the jigsaw, eventually contributing to a more accurate and realistic view of the whole picture (McFarlane and Harvey 2012).

INTRODUCTION

WHAT ARE THE ISSUES?

The issues and presenting behaviour:
Research findings from an inner-city arts project

Most of today's educators are finding that successful academic progress and healthy social-emotional development are intrinsically interwoven. A programme to look at the social and emotional aspects of learning (SEAL) has recently been rolled out across schools in the UK (LGfL 2011) and has proved very effective, not only in the UK but also in Australia and the USA.

In 2001 an experiment was conducted in an inner city in the UK, looking at the effectiveness of psychodynamic intervention in helping prevent school exclusions. Four art and dramatherapists worked across the city in six schools and, of the 124 children seen, 76 per cent were assessed by teachers to have shown signs of improvement as a result of the intervention. Another evaluation with eight therapists in ten schools in 2005 gave similar percentage results. The research results from their own work showed the therapists that the main issues facing the children they supported were neglect, domestic violence, parental separation, bullying, attachment and abuse with the presenting behaviours of anger, anxiety, stress and problems relating to low self-esteem. This book deals with the above issues as well as some less common occurrences such as bereavement, sibling rivalry and compulsive lying.

HOW CAN WE RECOGNIZE THE ISSUES?

Presenting behaviours: Classroom and playground

A key factor in looking at children's behaviour that may present as worrying has, for me, always been associated with a change, especially if there is no obvious cause. A child who has recently lost a significant member of the family is probably going to demonstrate some sort of difficult behaviour as is the child whose parents have recently separated. Similarly, a child whose primary role models persistently display violence and anger is likely to continue to react in an aggressive way to minor provocation no matter what intervention is introduced. With these children it is a matter of appropriate support and hopefully, in time, some sort of understanding and acceptance of their situations will alleviate their negative reactions and behaviour.

When a change in behaviour occurs for no apparent reason, it can become much more worrying and troublesome for staff. A child who previously has been outgoing becomes withdrawn, a hitherto easy-going child starts to have tantrums or aggressive outbursts or there is a sudden refusal or reluctance either to come to school or to go home: all these behaviours are trying to tell us that something is not right.

The question is – what? And how can we find out? Speaking as a children's therapist I do not underestimate the child's assessment of a situation, nor can I over-emphasize a child's ability to communicate that assessment through the medium of metaphor, in story, mime or play (see 'Metaphor and symbol', pp.32–33). However, although an interpretation of this communication should always remain the province of the trained therapist, it does not prevent the non-therapist from looking at the child from a different angle and asking the question, 'What is this behaviour trying to tell me?'

For example, in the case of a child who has suddenly become school phobic, it might be worthwhile, instead of simply presuming that it is the coming to school that is worrying the child, to ask the question, 'What is it that the child is afraid will happen at home if he is not there?' In the case of a child who has, through bereavement or other trauma, recently lost one parent, the anxiety may be that while he is at school, the other parent may disappear. A few years ago I dealt with the case of a child who had become school phobic because a member of the family was abusing her mother. While the child was at home, this could not and did not happen. In such cases it is always worth asking yourself, what does this behaviour serve to maintain?

Suggestions for assessment

In busy schools it is always difficult to find the time to find the reasons behind a child's behaviour, yet, in my opinion, it is paramount that we do so. Moreover, simply asking the question 'Why?' rather than dealing with what is seen as the bad behaviour may save time in the long run. Obviously, schools are not mini social services and many will say it is not their place to sort out what is happening to a child outside the school environment. Yet it is well documented that disaffected and emotionally unstable children cannot and do not progress well academically, so somehow a middle ground must be found.

However, if we ask a child the direct question, 'Why are you behaving like this?', we are very likely to get a shrug from an older child and a blank look from a younger. The simple truth is, often, they do not know or, if they do, they won't tell. Although it is not the job of school staff to act as detective agencies, it is helpful to be able to rule out certain explanations or at least pin the possible answers down to a general area.

With this in mind, in the case of a younger child who does not know, it is useful to be able to talk through the medium of a puppet. With an older child who will not say, the trick is not to pry and to use a displacement activity (see 'General and differentiated approaches', pp.28–29).

THE MAGIC THUMB

For younger children a simple technique that I have found to be effective is to use the 'magic thumb'. I explain to the child that when the thumb is at the top, then everything is fantastic: it couldn't be better. However, when it is at the bottom, everything is really bad and couldn't get worse. I start at the bottom and the child says, 'Stop' when he feels the 'magic thumb' is telling me where he is emotionally. If appropriate, I may then ask, 'What would make the thumb go up to the top?'

Very often the reply is something like, 'If I had a new computer game!', but occasionally this question results in a surprisingly helpful answer.

Most children seem to enjoy this activity and, in my experience, it has proved a reasonably accurate assessment of their emotional state, especially if is used over a period of a few weeks.

THE TRUTH GAME

Another useful exercise is to turn the question, 'What's wrong?' into a game. I explain that, if the child likes, we could play a guessing game. I say I know that not everything is okay (the thumb is not at the top) and I invite him to stand opposite me, a few paces away, and I will make some guesses as to what his troubles are about. I say there is one rule and that is that we always have to tell the truth. If I am right he has to take a step towards me and if I am wrong he can take a step away. If he reaches the door/wall/table, etc. then he has won, but if he reaches me, then I have won. In this way, by not looking at the child directly but talking rather to his position in the room, the focus is taken off the child, which enables him to relax.

I start with some outlandish guesses that are obviously not going to be right and may make him laugh before homing the questions into 'This is something to do with school/home/friends, etc.' Thus prompted the child will often then say what is wrong but it is helpful information even if the trouble is only pinned down to a general area: bullying at school, for example, or worry about mum going into hospital. Another way of approaching this issue, which puts the whole game on to a more equal footing, is to say that you can both make guesses about each other. This takes the intensity out of the situation and has the effect of normalizing the problem.

Severe case scenarios

During my time as a teacher and dramatherapist I have come across an alarming number of children whose level of behaviour warranted inclusion in a special school or unit but who, for one reason or another, were still being held in a mainstream school. The basic premise is usually that immediate referral to children's mental health services or other appropriate professional organizations is necessary, *if the child is a danger to himself or others.*

However, if for whatever reason a school finds itself having to hold such a child, then there are certain basic requirements and a minimum knowledge base necessary to be able to do so as safely as possible under the circumstances.

- Behaviour which gives cause for concern is a sudden switch from normal to agitated, frenzied and occasionally repetitive action, often accompanied by a rise in temperature and, in severe cases, profuse sweating. Staff have been known to comment that the child 'didn't seem himself' or was 'out of himself'. Eyes may be staring, darting from one side to the other or unfocused. The child is often unaware of what he is doing.

- Sometimes, but not always, the child may regress to behaving like a young child or toddler. In itself this is not alarming as many children behave this way to gain attention but it is the frenzied actions and/or level of focused concentration over a period of time (almost as if the child is remembering something) which may give cause for concern.

- With such behaviour it is necessary to avoid the 'triggers'. A consistently secure, familiar environment with known boundaries where the child can feel safe is desirable. So too is the designation of a member of staff who is able to be there for the child on all occasions. It is helpful if it is the same member of staff since the child will then be able to build up a level of trust that is so difficult to achieve with such damaged children. It is also worthwhile remembering that, in extreme cases, the child may view this member of staff as 'his' and may become violently jealous if forced to share the attention.

- If, despite all efforts to avoid the triggers, the child is overcome by an episode of alarming behaviour (I use the word 'overcome' advisedly since this is often how it appears), then it is important for the member of staff concerned to be aware of the following:

  - Make sure the child cannot escape from the room.

  - Take all potentially dangerous objects out of the child's reach and soften any hard areas with cushions or material.

  - Do not enter any fantasy or enactment except to say 'We can leave this baby/little one in a safe place now...'

  - Keep the voice, calm, controlled and kind but very firm.

  - Encourage the child to enter into another game or state of play (songs, rhymes or play that involves some sense of rhythm are usually the most effective).

  - When the child has calmed down or come out of the 'episode', use a calming technique to help restore normal behaviour (see 'Closure activities', pp.143–145 and 'Calming activities', pp.145–148). Sometimes it is helpful if the child keeps a list of his favourite techniques so that he can be in control of the choice, and hence his own behaviour.

WHAT CAN WE DO ABOUT THE ISSUES?
General and differentiated approaches

During my career of working first as a teacher, and then as a dramatherapist focused on developing children's emotional stability, I have found that the single most valuable technique to support children with emotional and behavioural problems is *to take time to enter their world*. By this I mean to really start where they are emotionally, not where you think they are or should be, as in the following example.

When I arrived to see Kevin at his primary school he was sitting outside his classroom. He had refused to go back in after lunchtime and had subsequently turned his back (literally) on any attempt to engage him, even in fun activities. When I walked in he was busy picking the balls of fluff off the chair covers in the corridor. I deposited my bag of games/ toys/material and watched him for a few minutes. He didn't look up.

Kneeling down at some distance from him, I began to copy him. For some minutes we remained happily engaged in picking fluff off our separate chairs. Then, without looking at him I began to line up my balls of fluff on the top of the chair and one by one I flicked them so that they rolled down the back. If they managed to reach the bottom I acknowledged the success with a loud 'Yes!'. Somewhat startled, Kevin turned to look at me. I ignored him.

Intrigued, Kevin slowly got up and took a few paces towards me to see what I was actually doing. I continued to ignore him. He went back to his own chair and began to copy me. Without looking at him I said, 'Shall we have a race?', and saw, out of the corner of my eye, that he nodded.

It very soon became obvious that a competition was impossible from our separate chairs and Kevin very happily agreed to share one. After focusing on the game for a little while it became an easy next step to start taking things out of my kitbag, and before long we were both engaged in playing with the puppets. There was no way Kevin would ever have entertained doing this half an hour before.

This displacement technique of pretending to be interested in something other than the child often works well with older children since, having reached the self-conscious age, it focuses the attention away from them and their problems. An example of this technique is given in the 'Through the Wall' story when a girl became engaged in spite of herself through my, not altogether fabricated, dismay over some broken glass animals (see McFarlane 2005).

With younger children, talking through the medium of a puppet often works well. A trick I have learnt is to say that the puppet does not want to talk to me and will only speak to the child. Thus, when I ask the question of the puppet, 'Why are you feeling so angry today?', the puppet will only tell the child the answer. Most children find this refusal to speak to me hugely entertaining, at least at first.

Just occasionally a child's behaviour will be highly symbolic of their undisclosed situation. A little girl whose family had just been bereaved began to spend her entire time at school hiding under a table. The truth was that at home it was an unspoken rule not to speak about or in any way acknowledge the death. The whole family was 'hiding' from the truth. In another scenario a little boy, who was being pulled in two different directions by his estranged parents and having to spend different nights each week at various houses, began to have temper tantrums in which he became a lion. He was being 'split' in so many ways that he himself was splitting or finding another personality that could cope with the changes. Since his name was Lionel, a lion was an obvious choice.

Since children are, on the whole, uncomplicated beings, sometimes the most uncomplicated and literal explanation for their behaviour is nearest the truth.

A child's concept of reality

In order to be able to understand what may be going on inside a child's head, which is affecting his behaviour, it may be useful to consider how a child's concept of reality differs from that of an adult. Here it is important to remember that it is not always the child's *chronological* age that we have to take into account. Depending on factors such as genetic, environmental, cultural and, most particularly, emotional (that is to say, the degree of subjection to emotional trauma) a child may have developed psychologically at a much slower, or sometimes, faster rate. A trained therapist will sometimes have to take a child back to the stage of development which was arrested by some emotional trauma, allowing him to play through relating issues and progress to the next stage in his own time. In my experience there is often a surprising correlation between outside events in a child's life and his stage of emotional development, as in the case of a little boy proclaimed by the mental health team to have a developmental delay of two years. Later we learnt from his mother that her divorce had meant that she had suffered with severe depression for two years.

Although we expect very little children to be literal in their concept of reality, it is also worthwhile remembering that a developmental delay may mean that an older child may view the world in this way too. This may give rise to all sorts of misunderstandings and feelings of guilt, confusion or anxiety. An 11-year-old girl with whose family I was working on bereavement issues presented as more withdrawn and anxious than could be readily understood. After some sessions it turned out that she thought her father, who had suffered a heart attack, had actually been attacked in his heart. She had not wanted to see him, blaming him for her parents' separation, and therefore thought that it was all her fault that he had died. 'If I had gone and told him how much I loved him, his heart wouldn't have been attacked and he wouldn't have died,' she told me.

Children on the Asperger's or autistic spectrum are more likely to view the world in this literal way and to make connections that are not always apparent to adults. Mary, a little girl with autistic traits who I was supporting, began to present with very difficult behaviour when her mother became pregnant. Everyone drew pictures of babies and explained to her what a lovely present this was going to be but she continued to refuse to leave her mother in the mornings and to have temper tantrums in class. Eventually, after many sessions we found out what was bothering her. Being profoundly deaf she had had to go to hospital many times for various operations. She had also visited her grandfather there just before he died. She associated hospitals as places where people had pain and died. Since there were complications with this pregnancy, her mother had to pay frequent visits to hospital, which she did without her daughter. The next time she went for a routine, pleasant check-up, we suggested that Mary went too.

Another aspect that is often overlooked in dealing with the way that children view the world is the fact that they are inclined to consider that everything revolves around them and cannot exist unless they are a part of it. This is not for selfish or self-centred reasons but rather because they may still be focused in, or developing from, that stage of development which is unable to separate themselves from others (see 'Stages of development', pp.33–34). For example, children often blame themselves for their parents' separation. I have had children saying to me, 'If I had kept my bedroom tidy my parents would still be together,' or, 'It was all my fault because mum and dad had to get a babysitter in for me.'

Seeing the world through a child's eyes is not always possible. I have, however, found it helpful, when considering the 'why?' of the behaviour, to try to remember that, on the whole, children still live in a world where anything is possible and that their experiments with the 'what ifs?' can sometimes lead them into making connections and imaginings totally alien to our adult, more reasoning and rational minds. Sometimes then too the violence of their behaviour will mirror the violence of their imaginary world in an effort to paint a realistic portrayal of their fears.

Fact and fantasy

We have already discussed the fact that, for very young children, the boundaries between fact and fantasy may become blurred and that, in their world, anything may be possible. Being able to enter into this land of make believe with a child, while at the same time keeping open the pathways back into the real world, helps him develop a healthy recognition of what is (as my daughter termed it) 'true life' and what is not. Mooli Lahad, founder and Director of the Institute of Dramatherapy, argues that although the boundaries may blur, young children *are* able to distinguish between fantasy and reality. He cites the example of a child who turns a chair into a horse and knows if it is trotting or galloping, but when a parent offers to feed it, will quickly (and often scornfully) rejoin with the fact that it is 'only a chair' (Lahad 2000, p.12). Unfortunately, many children are either not encouraged in this sort of healthy playacting or are subjected to too many conflicting messages to be able to differentiate between fact and fantasy. The world where anything not only can, but does, happen is then a very scary place.

An example of this is when a child is not only allowed to watch films and play computer games that are violent but is also subjected to witnessing domestic violence. It is no use telling such a child that these things only happen in films. He knows otherwise. However, what he does not know and cannot identify is whether the horrific events, which he has seen on film, are going to happen in real life. His inability to conceptualize abstract thought (see 'Metaphor and symbol', pp.32–33) adds to his confusion of what is real and what is not. All he knows is that the feeling of horror and fear which he experiences when watching the film and which is perpetrated by the scary people or monsters is the same feeling he gets when he witnesses violence at home. If the feelings are the same, then who is to say that the scary monsters won't attack him in his home?

A child who is caught in this world of confusion may often be thought of as a compulsive liar and work may need to be done to help him sort out in his head what is fact and what is fiction (see 'Compulsive lying', pp.87–91).

Underpinnings of dramatherapy
Metaphor and symbol

This next section attempts to give the background to the reasons for the choices of the activities and exercises in this book as well as to serve as an introduction to those not already familiar with the importance of metaphor and symbol in a child's play.

The developmental psychologist and philosopher Jean Piaget explained that children under a certain age find it very difficult to process abstract ideas (Piaget 1970). A small child can only understand the concept of death when he sees a dead bird or his hamster dies. Beauty and goodness are personified in fairy tales by the princess, magic by the fairy godmother and evil by the wicked witch.

Interestingly, this is still the way our subconscious sometimes works in dreams, which can use metaphors and symbols in a surprisingly literal way. Being 'let down' by a friend in real life may translate itself in a dream into being dropped by the friend from a high building, for example. Struggling up a hill may indicate real life upward battles and drowning may be trying to keep your head above water.

It is through this language of metaphor in his play that a young child will often communicate. It is much easier for him to tell you that the baby tortoise was unhappy because he couldn't run as fast as his friend the cheetah than try to explain the complex feelings he has around the fact that he is not as bright or as quick as his older brother and is afraid his parents do not love him as much. It doesn't take a trained therapist to be able to find ways to explore how a tortoise may not be quick but he has other attributes: for example, that he will always get there in the end, and that he carries his place of safety with him!

The exploration of a simple metaphor like this, if done purely to raise the child's self-esteem, can be safely embarked on since many children's books and stories already do just that. What should remain the province of the therapist is the intentional exploitation of more complicated metaphorical and symbolic situations that may involve an enactment of particular scenarios so that some sort of realization, acknowledgement and eventual healing can take place.

Stages of development: Embodiment, projection and role

The dramatherapeutic methodology which underpins the inclusion of many of the exercises and activities in this book can be attributed to a process called 'embodiment, projection and role' which roughly follows the stages of child development as outlined by psychological theorists J. Piaget (1970) and E.H. Erikson (1959). There are many other models of dramatherapy but this particular process is part of the Creative Expressive Model as invented by Sue Jennings (Jennings 1994) and is the one that I have found most useful in my work supporting children with emotional and behavioural problems in schools.

The 'embodiment' stage of development corresponds approximately to Piaget's 'sensory motor' stage and Erikson's 'trust versus mistrust' and is the stage in which the child is still totally absorbed by himself and his own physical needs. It is during this stage that a child first becomes aware of himself and this journey of self-exploration, and awareness can be supported by the arts or playtherapist through play with materials such as clay, sand, water, soft toys and brightly coloured material.

It is during the 'projection' stage that, according to Piaget, the child becomes aware of the world outside himself. Toys and other objects take on significance and can be used in therapy to represent extensions of family, friends or the child himself. Talking through the medium of a puppet (see 'General and differentiated approaches', pp.28–29) is a good example of the way a child can project his own feelings on to an inanimate object. In the adult world we come across projection when we attribute others with the faults and failings of which we ourselves are guilty.

The age at which children will progress through these stages will depend on a variety of factors, not least the degree to which they have been subjected to emotional trauma (see 'Trauma and shock', pp.139–141). As a rough guide, a child will begin to go through the projective stage after the age of two and will begin to be able to use role from the age of about seven.

It is during the 'role stage' that, according to Piaget, a child begins to be able to understand others' points of view and to see himself as others see him. Erikson suggests that this stage is when a child becomes aware of his own identity as opposed to the other confusing roles he is forced to play. It is the job of the drama or other arts therapist to encourage the child to develop, through role-play, a healthy repertoire of roles that will enable him to interact, as far as possible, in a functional rather than dysfunctional way, with members of his family and wider society (Landy 1993). Thus it is that, through role-play, a child can explore various 'what if?' situations to discover what behaviours and roles have the most promising outcomes in a kind of 'rehearsal for life' scenario.

Dramatic distancing

A technique employed by dramatherapists is that of dramatic distancing in which a fictional character is created onto which the feelings of the child are projected (see 'Parental separation', pp.115–122). In this way the feelings can be viewed objectively as if through the wrong end of a telescope and this distancing can allow the child the emotional space and safety to be more reasoning and less reactive.

Directive and non-directive intervention

A premise underpinning my work as a dramatherapist and which has a bearing on the activities presented in this book is the extent to which the intervention, or in this case, support for the child, is directive or non-directive. That is to say, how much do you let the child control the sessions and how much do you direct him to follow your lead? With a child who has been subjected to abuse or overbearing adult behaviour, the issue of control is a big one (see 'Abuse', pp.42–48), and this should always be borne in mind when dealing with any child with emotional and behavioural problems. As a dramatherapist I would always employ non-directive intervention to allow the child to bring to me the issues on which he wanted to work before setting the appropriate stage on which he could act to bring about his own healing.

However, since this book is not intended to be used in a therapeutic way, or with children who need that level of input, the support as outlined in the activities can be more directive in nature, providing the above considerations concerning control are taken into account.

Using drama techniques

Show, don't tell

Using drama techniques for emotional support can be very effective but it can also be intensely stimulating for the child concerned. It is for this reason that the advice given in the specific activities should always be followed and care taken to ensure the child returns to his normal activities in a calm and controlled way, following what may have been a period of unsettled emotions.

On the whole what we are dealing with when we use action rather than verbal techniques in emotional support is to be found in the difference between the right and left hemispheres of the brain. The use of psychodrama to treat trauma survivors is becoming increasingly recommended as a 'viable treatment alternative' and 'many of the symptoms are unconscious, non-verbal right-brained experiences that cannot in fact be accessed through talk therapy' (Kellerman and Hudgins 2000, p.12). Although we are not dealing here with issues as severe as post-traumatic stress, the premise is still applicable to less emotionally damaging situations. In other words, just talking about an emotionally powerful experience is not always enough.

On the other hand, there is a huge danger in re-enacting a particular situation (unless specific training in dramatherapy or psychodrama has been undertaken) for fear of re-traumatization. *That is why it is paramount that a child never plays himself in any re-enactment but that this is always done through the dramatic distancing of a fictional character* (see 'Parental separation', pp.115–122).

The following are brief explanations of the drama techniques referred to later in the Activities section.

Deroling   After any enactment it is very important that a child comes out of role completely before he returns to the classroom or playground, especially if he has been playing a negative role such as a bully. A way to achieve this is to ask the child to take off the character as if he were taking off a coat and throw it down while saying 'I am not [the character]. I am [his name].' With longer enactments or especially in cases where the child would benefit from differentiating between the positive and negative traits of his character, the following procedure can be adopted.

Place two chairs side by side. Invite the child to sit in one as his character and talk about what positive traits he would like to keep from this character and which negative ones he would like to throw away. Then ask him to derole as above, sit in the other chair and talk about how it felt to play that character.

Doubling   This technique involves a hand being placed on the shoulder of the person playing that character to encourage him to say how he feels.

Note of caution: This should be restricted to a single word or phrase.

Freeze frames   Useful in a group situation when a scene from a story needs to be depicted. A way of introducing these is to suggest obvious scenes such as a wedding, christening or a scene from a well-known fairy tale. The group arranges themselves into the tableau, paying particular attention to facial expressions and body language and then 'freezes'.

Hot seating   To 'flesh out' a character, other members of the group can fire questions at a volunteer who is sitting in the 'hot seat'. The volunteer must then answer these questions without thinking too much, which usually results in the character being more authentic.

Mirroring   Usually done in pairs, this involves one person copying in minute details the actions, gestures, expressions or body language of the other person.

Reframing   This addresses the need to leave any enactment on a positive note by replacing a negative or destructive memory with a more pleasant one. It can be done by simply re-enacting the scene and changing body language, speech and facial expressions accordingly.

Role reversal	If done in a light-hearted manner this can be effective in helping a child to understand what it is like to be in another's shoes or how he might appear to others. The procedure is simply to swap roles with him and play through or mirror his role or body language so that he can see it from an objective point of view.
Sculpting	For individuals or groups, this technique involves moulding the body into a position that shows the feelings and can also involve facial expressions. With a group it can also incorporate the relative positions of the group members to describe their different relationships. A way to introduce this is to see if a group can guess from the body language how one of its members is feeling.
Speaking from role	Sometimes much insight can be gained not only by the group but also by the child in character if he is asked questions by the group and answers them in role. For example, a child playing the bully may be asked what was really making him angry and may answer that he himself was being bullied.

ACTIVITIES

WHAT TO DO AT THE BEGINNING OF A SESSION
Introductory exercises

Most children like routine and if their world is, on the whole, chaotic, the more structured the sessions, the safer they will feel. Starting a session in the same or similar way each week is therefore a good idea and allows progression from the familiar to the unfamiliar in a measured way. Some sort of check-in process is also advisable, especially if the child is being monitored over a period of weeks.

BEST AND WORST

Suggestions for this might be 'The Magic Thumb' (see 'Suggestions for assessment', pp.25–26) or 'Best and Worst' which involves inviting the child to think of the best thing to have happened to him during the past week followed by the worst. Offering your own examples first may make the exercise easier. This is designed to help the child on the first steps towards building emotional literacy and identifying different emotions.

USING RITUAL FOR TRANSITION PURPOSES

Depending on the child and his level of engagement and enjoyment in imaginary processes another possible introduction to a session might be to mark the transition between the everyday world of reality and the world of imaginative play in some way. This is also recommended for those children who have had little or no experience of being encouraged in their play, those for whom, very often, play means passively sitting in front of a television or computer screen (see 'Fact and fantasy', pp.31–32). Such children will often require a gentle welcoming into this world of fascinating and explorative fantasy and marking this with a ritual that becomes familiar over the weeks will support this transition. A suggested routine might be to use stepping-stones made out of cushions or material, a small tent or magic carpet which flies away to another land. Whichever medium is used, it is important to remember to repeat the process in reverse when returning to the world of reality. Equally, it is important for the child to know that, in this imaginary place, the 'what ifs?' of life can be safely explored but that they are left behind on returning to everyday reality (see 'Compulsive lying', pp.87–91).

Group warm-up games

Whereas the above introductory exercises are as applicable to a group as to individuals, a number of children may require additional warm-up activities to help them function as a group. These would normally involve some sort of physical exercise, eye contact and trust building games (see the activities in 'Attachment', pp.58–65) as well as games or activities that focus on the group working together. Suggestions for these are as follows.

Physical warm-ups

HULA HOOPS

- Invite the child or children to imagine they have a hula hoop. (What colour is it?)
- Tell them to start circling it on one wrist, then one arm.
- Ask them to fling it to the other wrist, then the arm.
- Repeat this with ankles, legs and finally the torso and waist.

PNEUMATIC DRILL

- Ask the children to stand in a circle and tell them that today they are road menders.
- Say they have in front of them a very large pneumatic drill with which they are going to drill a hole in the road.
- Invite them to pick it up and switch it on.
- Begin to make the noise of the drill and show the vibration running from the hands through the whole body.
- Invite them to copy you until everyone is shaking all over with the noise and vibration of the drill.
- Don't forget to switch off the drill at the end!

Group participation

CHANGING THE RHYTHM

–   Ask the group to sit in a circle.

–   Send one volunteer out of the room while you pick a child to change the rhythm.

–   The volunteer comes back into the room and stands in the centre of the circle while the group (following the designated child's lead) begins to clap hands, knees, thighs, etc. in rhythmic unison.

–   The child in the centre has to guess who is changing the rhythm.

COUNTING UP

–   Ask the children to stand in a circle as close together as possible. (This is best played with groups of not less than four and no more than 15.)

–   Say that you are going to count 1, 2, 3, 4, etc. together as a group, one after the other. If any two people say the same number the group must start back at '1' again.

–   Explain to the children that their best chance of success lies in doing this slowly and getting eye contact with each other to try to guess if they are about to say something.

Variation: The group members can take a step forward as they say a number. This has the effect of making it easier to guess who is about to speak and is therefore more useful with younger children.

This activity is a good gauge of how well the group is working together. It is also a valuable lesson to those who are inclined to push themselves forward at the expense of others.

ISSUES, BEHAVIOURS AND SUPPORTING ACTIVITIES

ABUSE

The issue

Since no book on offering emotional support to children would be complete without a section on abuse, I am including a short synopsis of what might be helpful in terms of what constitutes abuse and, more particularly, what behaviours in the child should give cause for alarm and what might be considered normal. Having said this, any causes for concern, no matter how slight, should always be discussed with whoever is responsible for child protection since, although they may not be noteworthy in themselves, they may contribute to a disturbing pattern or overall picture.

According to the National Society for the Prevention of Cruelty to Children (NSPCC), from figures taken from the numbers of children on child protection registers or the subject of child protection plans, approximately 46,700 children in the UK were known to be at risk of abuse in March 2010. Furthermore, a survey carried out by the NSPCC in 2009 of young adults aged 18–24 showed that one in four had been severely maltreated during childhood (NSPCC 2011a).

Abuse in childhood is often categorized under three headings: physical, emotional and sexual, with the issue of severe neglect (see 'Neglect', pp.106–111) also raising child protection concerns.

Physical abuse may involve hitting, throwing, shaking, poisoning, burning, scalding, drowning, suffocating or in any other way causing physical harm to a child. Feigning the symptoms of, or deliberately causing ill health to a child, also constitutes physical abuse.

Emotional abuse is involved to some measure in all types of ill treatment of children but it may occur alone. Persistently conveying to a child that he is unloved, worthless, inadequate or undervalued to the extent that this has severe adverse effects on his emotional development constitutes emotional abuse. So too does the exploitation or corruption of children, putting them in constant danger or continually causing them to feel frightened or having expectations of them which are totally inappropriate for their age.

Sexual abuse is defined as the forcing, enticing or encouragement of a child to take part in sexual activities whether or not they involve contact and whether or not the child is aware of what he is doing. These activities may range from full penetrative sex to watching or being exposed to pornographic films and videos or being encouraged to behave in a sexually inappropriate way.

The behaviours

A change in the 'normal' behaviour pattern of a child can be a key indicator that there may be a cause for concern. Having said this, there may well be other issues going on for the child and it is necessary to distinguish between what is indisputable fact (and make a written note of it) and what is opinion (yours or anyone else's). Investigation remains the responsibility of the appropriate authorities that can only collate and act on written evidence.

Areas for concern

Physical abuse in terms of injuries suffered by a child can vary considerably from one child to another. Some children seem to have a habit of falling over or having accidents. Diagnosis of physical abuse is difficult since, from the appearance of the injury, it is rarely absolutely clear whether it has been inflicted or is purely accidental. Some sites of injury or particular situations raise more suspicions of child abuse than others. Although not a definitive list, these may include the following:

- Injuries sustained by a baby or child not yet toddling.
- Injury to the inside of arms or inside or back of legs, ears, eyes, buttocks or genitals.
- Bruises that reveal the imprint of a hand, fist, belt or other instrument.
- Delay in obtaining medical attention or offering no explanation for injury.
- Cigarette burns, scalds or other burns that may indicate a child being forced near to a hot object. (Difficult to diagnose since these may be merely skin infections.)

Emotional abuse is perhaps the most difficult to diagnose since children experience widely different standards of care. Some forms of emotional abuse may include the following:

- Extreme over-indulgence or over-protection to the extent that the child is emotionally inhibited.
- Persistent, excessive (and often public) belittling, sarcasm and ridicule.
- Encouraging hostility from others including other children.
- Excessive teasing that has a frightening or threatening edge.
- Persistent scapegoating or making the child the odd one out in the family.
- Excessive emotional downloading that is age-inappropriate.
- Subjection to deprivation of basic needs or promising treats and constantly reneging.

Sexual abuse is an emotive subject and is often fraught with difficulty in terms of assessing what is normal and what should be considered abnormal behaviour. In short it is normal for young, growing children to want to explore their own sexual parts and those of others, especially of the opposite sex. The playing of doctors and nurses or mummies and daddies by four- and five-year-olds is normal behaviour as is rubbing themselves when they are tired or before falling asleep. What is not normal is if the role-play contains any persistent coercion on the part of one child towards another that may indicate a replay of abuse. The following are behaviours that constitute a cause for concern and should be noted and referred appropriately:

- Frequent rubbing of genitals instead of playing.
- Simulation of the act of intercourse.
- Always wanting to watch adults dressing or undressing or in the bathroom.
- Unnatural and persistent curiosity about sex.
- Forcing other children to play doctors, for example, undressing, exploring each other.

- Persistent hinting of a secret they cannot tell or seeming to have a secret they cannot tell or a friend with a problem.

- Suddenly starting bed wetting for no apparent medical reason (especially if coupled with nightmares).

- Beginning to lie, cheat or steal in the hope of being caught.

- Having sudden inexplicable changes of behaviour such as becoming very withdrawn or aggressive or suddenly developing an eating disorder such as anorexia or bulimia.

- Having a poor self-image or starting to self-harm.

- Becoming severely depressed, threatening or attempting suicide.

Activity

It is not my intention to include within this section any activities expressly aimed at supporting the abused child since that must remain the province of the trained therapist. Rather, the following activity concentrates on increasing self-esteem and confidence by allowing the child not only to be in control but also to feel protected, a situation that is the direct antithesis of abuse.

Note of caution: Although it is paramount that children who are suffering from abuse receive professional therapeutic support, this is usually considered inadvisable while the abuse is ongoing. In other words, as a matter of priority the child must be in a safe place before therapy can be effective. Although the following exercise is not therapeutic in nature I would still advise that any enactment be avoided if abuse is suspected to be ongoing.

THE SHIELD

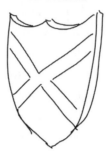

Resources

A3 or A2 card
Coloured pens or crayons
Paints (optional)
Glue or string to fasten
Dressing-up clothes or lengths of material (optional)

Application

This exercise is most effective, at least initially, if used with an individual child so that he benefits from the undivided attention needed to help him re-establish a sense of self-esteem, power and control.

Objectives

Since a child who has been abused often suffers from a loss of sense of self, this exercise is aimed at helping him recreate a sense of who he is by recalling and putting into concrete form details about himself and his life. By looking at future events it also reassures him that there is a chance that things will get better. Additionally it builds a metaphorical protection mechanism around the child by reminding him of who is there to help him. The subsequent use of the shield in overcoming monsters is directed towards putting the child back into a place of control over his life.

> *Note of caution: Any subsequent enactment should be at the child's instigation, with the child remaining in control and directing the nature and level of 'nastiness' of the monster. This enactment should remain entirely in the metaphor and should bear no resemblance whatsoever to the original abuse. If there is any danger of this being the case it should be stopped immediately and a calming exercise introduced (see 'Severe case scenarios', pp.26–27 and 'Calming activities', pp.145–148).*

Exercise

- With the child (or as a prior activity), cut out the shape of a large shield from the card. You may also wish to cut an oblong length for an armband (or string may be used instead).
- Divide the shield into five sections and label each as follows: What I'm going to be when I grow up, Where I'm going to live when I grow up, What I like doing and am good at (if this is difficult restrict to 'like doing'), My friends, People who help me.
- Invite the child to write or draw in each section.
- The shield can then be decorated around the edge in favourite colours, with favourite cartoon characters, football teams, fairies, stars, butterflies, rainbows, etc. (All shapes and colours should be light, bright and positive.)
- An armband can then be attached (from top to middle) so that the shield can be worn.

Extension

The aim with this subsequent enactment is to encourage the child to use his shield in an active way so that he gains a sense of having something, which he has made himself and which is an extension of himself, constantly available as a form of protection. In a sense he has externalized a stronger more positive part of himself that can protect the more vulnerable 'inner child'.

With the provisos above, the shield can then be used to overcome 'monsters'. This enactment could be prefaced by the words, 'I expect you feel really strong when you're wearing this. I'd be really scared if I was a monster.'

The child can then be encouraged to brandish his shield and fight off any foes. The whole enactment should be kept on the level of a light-hearted, mock play battle.

Further activities

Activities that help to raise a child's self-esteem and confidence and encourage him to stand up for himself are useful here (see 'Lack of self-esteem/confidence', pp.96–102 and 'Bullying', pp.75–83).

Activities involving the building of trust are useful here especially for children for whom physical contact has not necessarily been a pleasant experience (see 'Attachment: Trust activities', pp.58–65).

Other issues addressed

Bereavement, bullying, depression, lack of self-esteem/confidence and neglect.

ANGER

The issue

A child who has a sudden temper tantrum is an all too frequent occurrence in the normal routine of a school and can be difficult to deal with unless the school has adequate provision to calm him down. By 'adequate' provision I mean a member of staff skilled enough to manage the often violent behaviour as well as a room safe enough to work in. Something that is often overlooked is the fact that angry, aggressive behaviour is the result of angry, aggressive emotions that in turn hide a deep sense of hurt and sadness usually associated on some level with loss. This can be the loss of a parent through bereavement or separation, the loss of trust in a relationship or set of circumstances, loss of self-esteem, confidence or identity through abuse or neglect or simply loss of faith or hope in the future. Whatever the loss, it can only be treated once the angry feelings have been dealt with.

Depending on the age of the child and the severity of the loss, this can take some time. In my experience whatever the child's age a worthwhile starting point is to consider ways in which to allow the child to express his anger in a safe way. In other words, *expression* rather than *repression* should be the underlying objective once requirements of 'understanding consequences' and 'sending out suitable messages to others' have been met. Any safe activities, therefore, which energetically meet the anger on an equal basis and which may become a catalyst for uncovering the hurt beneath should be considered. What is not helpful is to continually use repressive, confining activities without allowing the child a means of expressing the anger he already feels. These activities can include any action that involves letting go of energy inside, whether this be through extended breathing exercises, thumping a cushion or merely running ten times around the playground.

A less exhausting alternative, however, may be a small room that can be made safe and equipped with soft toys, cushions and lengths of coloured material. Many schools have found this provision of space invaluable when it comes to managing angry children. A child can then be invited to take part in various safe but cathartic activities before doing some form of relaxation, for example, creative visualization while listening to calming music, art or craft or simply breathing exercises. Anger management is usually most effective when both these activities, that is, the cathartic and relaxation, are used. Relaxation on its own will not work if the child is still feeling angry and exercises which discharge anger require a period of calm before the child can be safely returned to class.

The behaviours

Anger can manifest itself in a variety of behaviours ranging from tantrums to a cold, insular 'shutting off' demeanour. Margot Sunderland, in *The Science of Parenting* (2006), tells us that when a child is having a tantrum his brain is being flooded with extremely high levels of the stress hormone, cortisol. Left for prolonged periods this chemical can reach toxic levels that may damage a developing brain. A child who is in the throes of a tantrum or whose anger has spiralled out of control cannot talk or listen properly since these stress chemicals affect the centres for cognitive thought and verbal expression in his higher brain. Trying to reason with or talk a child out of an angry episode is therefore useless. All you can do is try to discharge the feelings that are too big for him to handle.

Sunderland differentiates between the 'higher and lower' brain, which, broadly speaking, refers to the rational, reasoning and primitive instinctual parts of the brain. It is the higher brain which, when properly developed, is able to calm and control the instinctual, raging emotions, those 'big feelings' which threaten to overwhelm a small child. In order for the higher brain to develop properly, consistent, emotionally supportive and responsive caring needs to take place. Then, healthy pathways between the higher and lower parts of the brain are forged and the child is able to monitor his emotions and feel empathy for others. Sunderland also tells us that brain scans show that many violent adults are still driven by the 'lower brain' since the 'higher brain' has not received the necessary stimuli for it to develop properly.

Areas for concern

A more worrying scenario is the child who does not outwardly display his anger but who appears coldly removed from any display of emotion. I remember working with a child such as this who described the angry feelings in his head as blue. This child had retreated so far into himself to avoid the damaging outside world that he was no longer able to 'feel' anything very much at all. In these instances carefully measured work needs to be done to encourage the child to get back in touch with his feelings, but this is work for the qualified therapist and should not be attempted without adequate training.

Another potentially referable situation is when, during an angry episode, a child's temperature rises to the extent that he sweats profusely. If this occurs repeatedly it may be evidence of a psychotic aspect underlying the anger and should be referred to the appropriate professional (see 'Severe case scenarios', pp.26–27).

Activities

MR. ANGRY MAN

Resources
Paper
Pencils, coloured pens

Application
This can be done with a small group but is more effective if used with an individual child. It is also applicable to other feelings such as anxiety, fear, panic, jealousy, etc. It is not suitable for a child who is in the throes of a tantrum but could be used with children who suffer from repeated angry episodes, when they are in a calm state of mind and able to reason.

Objectives
The aim of this exercise is to enable the child to feel in control of his 'big feelings' by externalizing them. That is to say that by personifying them, or making them into another person, the child can view them (or it) objectively and not become subjectively overwhelmed.

Exercise
 – Tell the child that you understand how he feels. Say that it's like there is a Mr. Angry Man who has a habit of sneaking up and taking over almost without him realizing what is happening.
 – Ask him if he would like to draw this Mr. Angry Man.

- When Mr. Angry Man has been drawn a dialogue can be instigated in which the child can tell Mr. Angry Man how fed up he is with him sneaking up and that he wants him to go away, etc.
- If applicable, a role-play exercise can be used in which the child rehearses a situation where Mr. Angry Man might sneak up. The drawing can then be used for the child to face Mr. Angry Man and tell him to 'go away'.
- Additionally, the process can be turned into a kind of game in which the child has to see if he can outwit Mr. Angry Man and banish him before he takes over.
- To help with this some breathing techniques can be used the minute the child feels Mr. Angry Man is about to pounce (see 'The Saucepan', pp.52–54 and 'Breathing techniques', pp.145–148).

THE VOLCANO

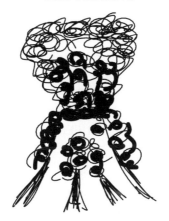

Resources
Lengths of coloured material
Cushions
A3 card
Coloured pens
Sticky paper

Application

This is useful as an energy releasing exercise but must be performed in an environment that is safe and free from sharp objects, for example, cornered tables, in case the child throws himself around excessively.

Objectives

The aim is to release the built-up energy of the emotion and this is more effective if done with an energy-releasing breathing exercise such as 'The Saucepan' (pp.52–54), followed by some calming activity.

Exercise

- Make a huge pile of cushions and material in the middle of the room.
- Tell the child that this is a volcano and that it is angry; in fact, it is boiling inside.
- Ask the child if he would like to get into the middle of the volcano to see how it feels.
- Pile the material on top of the child.
- Say the volcano is getting hotter and hotter and angrier and angrier. It will soon have to explode.
- Tell the child you will count back from ten. When you get to zero it will explode.
- Count back and allow the child to burst out from underneath the material and then fling it (like lava) around the room.
- The child may want to repeat this exercise. Allow him to repeat it as many times as it takes for him to feel calmer.

THE SAUCEPAN

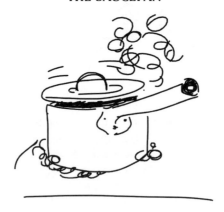

Resources
None

Application

This can be used in isolation as a way of releasing strong emotions through breathing or as a follow-up from a physical energy-release activity such as 'The Volcano'. Other examples of breathing techniques, in particular 'The Woodchopper' (pp.145–146), which also focuses on the release of pent-up energy, can be found in 'Calming activities' (pp.145–148).

Objectives

The objective is to give the child a captivating and easily-accessible image to help him release pent-up stress.

Exercise

– Talk to the child about how it feels to have all your feelings bottled up. Explain that it is rather like a saucepan in which potatoes (or equivalent) are being boiled.

– Ask the child what would happen if you put your hand over the lid and kept it there.

– Explain that this is what happens if we keep our feelings bottled up all the time and don't express them safely or a little bit at a time. (This explosion then usually gets us into trouble with teachers, parents, etc.)

– Mime taking the lid off the saucepan repeatedly, allowing the steam to escape safely a little at a time.

– Show the child how to take a deep breath in and then allow the breath to escape as you raise the saucepan lid.

– The last out-breath should be long as you keep the lid raised and allow the remainder of the breath to escape.

Extensions

Once the child has acted out being an angry volcano a sufficient number of times and has completed other energy-releasing exercises if necessary, he may be sufficiently calm and receptive enough to be able to reason and understand the source of his anger. Cognitive work can then be attempted such as drawing a big picture of a volcano and allowing the child to write, draw or place sticky paper on the volcano to depict the sort of things that make him angry. The things that make him a little angry can be placed at the bottom, moderately so in the middle but the potentially explosive situations should go at the top. In this way a child may be helped to understand the issues which really underlie his anger and how relatively unimportant happenings can be potentially explosive trigger points.

Further activities

'The Volcano' exercise is best attempted with an individual child. A group activity to release tension or anger might be to ask the children to imagine they are some kind of robotic or alien character that makes violent jerky movements. Allow them to play with this for a while and then ask them to swap to being a floppy rag doll. Alternating between these two states can reduce physical and emotional tension.

Activities that promote relaxation and calm are advised after tension and energy-release exercises. Guided visualizations with or without music and gentle breathing exercises are useful resources (see 'Calming activities', pp.145–148).

Other issues addressed

Anxiety, bereavement, bullying, parental separation and sibling rivalry.

ANXIETY

The issue

In looking at the issue of the anxious child in school it may be helpful first to consider what we mean by the term 'anxiety'. Broadly speaking, it belongs to that classification of psychological disorders called neuroses, which refers to the fact that, unlike psychoses, the patient is aware of the disturbance in their thinking and does not seek to fabricate a series of implausible reasons for their behaviour. The important fact to remember here is that a child who shows signs of a generalized anxiety, or even a monosymptomatic fear such as a phobia of some description, is aware *on some level* that their behaviour is not normal and wants to have help to change it.

Traditionally, anxiety was thought of as the result of early environmental disturbances, but more recently research has shown that there may also be some connection to chemical imbalances in the brain that may be alleviated by chemical input. Just as psychotherapy and cognitive behavioural therapy (CBT) have been known to help those adults suffering from states of anxiety, so play, creative arts therapy and behavioural support are often introduced to help the young child.

Although it goes without saying that overly anxious or phobic children should be referred to a specialist as a matter of course, the fact remains that, in practice, many such children remain for months on a waiting list while the school still has to manage their disturbing and sometimes disruptive behaviour.

In general then, the anxious child we meet in school may be suffering from what is commonly known as pervasive anxiety: this is a generalized over-activity of the nervous system which does not focus on one target (in which case it would be called a phobia). There is often (although this is difficult to establish) a history of neurosis in the family, but the most that can safely be said is that this may predispose a child to this condition. Very often there have been instances of distorted parental relationships such as over-protectiveness or there may have been experiences of separation from the primary carer. There may have been other initial anxiety-provoking events now difficult to identify because they have been either forgotten or repressed.

Sunderland (2006) speaks about the genetically ingrained emotional systems of rage, fear and stress that are deep within the lower brain. In the early years a child's developing brain is highly vulnerable to stress and (as we have seen with anger), when he is not adequately helped with his 'big feelings', the alarm systems in the lower brain can become over-active, resulting in over-reaction to minor stresses in later life. He may then grow up to be constantly 'on a short fuse' or live in a state of general anxiety. However, when a child's distress is met with adequately comforting responses, the chemicals of oxytocin and oproids (the feel-good factor) are released naturally in a child's brain and, together with the reasoning capability of a well-developed higher brain, help to quieten the clamouring alarm system of the lower brain.

The behaviours

In the light of research that has been done into the functioning of the brain, it would seem that a primary objective for staff in dealing with a child who is over-anxious or angry would be to try to help him deal with his 'big feelings'. Unfortunately, unlike the angry child (unless it is the cold anger described in 'Anger', pp.48–54), the anxious child is not always obvious by his behaviour. Night fears, bed wetting, nail biting and school phobia are outward signs of general anxiety disorder, but these may not be apparent at school or may be easily missed. Very often the first indication that there is anything wrong will come from home, and then it may be a difficult job for the school to unravel the sometimes very complex issue of where the anxiety originates and indeed, often, to whom it belongs!

The following points might be useful to remember when dealing with an anxious child.

- Has this child always been of an anxious nature and, if not, what was the trigger event? An interview with the parents may establish whether this has stemmed from a misunderstanding or whether indeed it is the parents' own anxiety filtering through to the child (both common in my experience).

- In the case of school phobia, what does it serve to maintain? What is the child frightened of that will happen if he is not at home? (This is common in cases of parental separation or bereavement when the child is frightened the other parent will disappear.)

- Has the child been having any recurring nightmares? These are often a clue to underlying chronic anxiety and may be addressed either directly or through the use of metaphors (see 'Nightmares', pp.111–115).

- Is the anxiety of such a severity that the child is showing signs of an altered state of awareness or suffering from a hugely curtailed quality of life? In either of these cases professional advice should be sought.

Activities

BEN'S BAG OF WORRIES

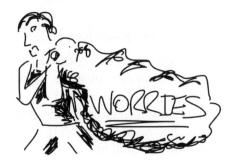

Resources

Small figures of characters or animals
Puppets
Paper
Coloured pens

Application and objectives

The primary objective here is to *externalize* the worry or anxiety into a shape or form to which the child can relate but which is not an integral part of him. In this way the worry can be reduced to a manageable size and is not seen as something that is taking over his life. Sometimes, however, a child is reluctant to explain the worry or does not know exactly why he is anxious, and then the following exercise may be useful.

Exercise

- Invite the child to make up a story with you about a little boy (or girl if the child is female).
- Say that you can use the little figures and ask him to choose a figure to be Ben (or whatever name you choose).
- Tell him that Ben has a big bag of worries and together you're going to make up a story about one of them.
- Use small figures (or puppets) to be other characters in the story.
- Don't comment on or try to direct the story. Allow the child to take the lead.
- Pay particular attention to whether Ben has anyone to help him with his worry and if not, at the end, ask if there was anyone Ben could have talked to who might have helped him.

Note: This story can remain completely in the metaphor and will be nonetheless supportive for the child (see 'Metaphor and symbol', pp.30–31). The child is projecting his own feelings on to another character, giving him a safe distance from which to explore them (see 'Stages of development', pp.33–34).

Extensions

Once the cause of the anxiety has been established it can sometimes be given a name and addressed in a playful fashion that reduces its impact on the child. This is especially useful in the case of a child with a mild phobia. *Note that severe phobic reactions require professional advice.* For example, a child who is afraid of being sick may wish to draw out this fear and then give it a name such as 'Icky'. A dialogue between the child and Icky can then take place with the child telling Icky he doesn't want him around and the whole scenario can then become a game of trying to catch Icky out before he sneaks up on the child (see 'Anger: Mr. Angry Man', p.48–54).

Further activities

Drawing out the 'big feelings' can be another way of externalizing issues for the child. Having big sheets of paper in separate corners of the room so that the child can draw out different emotions, for example, angry, sad, afraid, helps differentiate between these feelings. Being able to physically move between the areas of the room allows the child to separate out his emotions and understand the links between them (see 'Depression: Opposite Corners', pp.91–96).

Other issues addressed

Bullying, change or transition, lack of self-esteem/confidence, nightmares, parental separation, speech problems.

ATTACHMENT
The issue

Within this context attachment may be described as the need for the young child to cultivate a secure relationship with at least one primary carer in order to have a healthy social and emotional development. According to John Bowlby, originator of Attachment Theory and author of the informative book *Attachment and Loss* (1969), this need may have its origins in an evolutionary survival strategy that protected the small child from surrounding predators.

It is the child's fear of separation from a parent or carer in case something happens to him that can become (often incongruously) intense that poses problems, not only for the parent but also for the staff who are trying to assume care of the child. If, for some reason, this fear of separation has been allowed to grow out of proportion during the first few months and years of life then the child will have developed what is known as an 'insecure attachment'.

So what does a 'secure attachment' look like? It works both ways. In a secure attachment not only will the parent have met the child's needs but the child will also have met the parent's needs. The child will feel that their primary care giver is responsive, that there is nothing to fear and that he can therefore give himself permission to respond to other stimuli, developing a sound understanding of social situations and empathy with others. He will have developed a coherent and organized state of mind and an ability to regulate his own emotions. The parent will recognize that his or her own efforts at parenting have been well received and will continue to respond in a loving way. Secure attachment brings with it a healthy development of the higher human brain, which will help the child in later life access compassion, reflection and negotiation.

At the opposite end of the scale, neglect and abuse can have such severe effects on the developing brain at critical periods of growth as to block the release of hormones important to our feelings of wellbeing (see 'Anxiety', pp.54–58). In addition, if a child is not adequately comforted during times of severe reaction to his state of anger or anxiety then the stress hormone cortisol is produced which has an additional damaging effect on the brain (see 'Anger', pp.48–54). If the attachment is not secure, any of the systems linked with attachment in the lower brain such as rage, fear, distress, seeking and care can be activated, producing intense feelings which can continue into adulthood.

The behaviours

The ability to form attachments has been divided into four different patterns – secure, insecure/ambivalent, insecure/avoidant and insecure/ disorganized.

A key characteristic of the 'insecure/ambivalent' pattern is unpredictability, when the child is never sure how his parent will react and therefore does not know how to behave in order to bring about the desired reaction. The parent, preoccupied with self, may be deceptive, fail to keep promises or be inconsistently available and the child may switch from angry to charming or desperate, becoming clingy and, in later life, over-dependent on others or resorting to drugs or violence.

The 'insecure/avoidant' pattern is the avoidance of shows of emotion, which may result in feelings being 'shut down' or suppressed in later life. The parent is unresponsive to the child's distress and encourages the child to be self-reliant to the extent that he may become compulsively so or may develop a compulsive caring attitude to others and/or anger towards himself.

In an 'insecure/disorganized' pattern a child may experience his parent as either frightened or frightening. If the former, the child will constantly check facial expressions to make sure the situation is a safe one. If the parent appears frightening, this will place the child in a dilemma insofar as this primary care giver is at the same time a source of safety and of alarm. The child may then experience human interactions as erratic, and be unable to develop an organized and coherent behaviour pattern himself.

Different types of attachment disorder behaviours might be running and hiding, using promiscuous language and conduct, psychosomatic symptoms (physical ailments produced by psychological stress), inhibited (finding it very difficult to ask somebody for help) and hypervigilant (constantly being on the alert).

Activities

Since the issue of attachment involves primary care givers it is difficult to suggest any specific activities that might adequately address this in isolation (that is, a member of staff supporting the individual child). Some organizations have enlisted the help of play therapists to work with parents and children in the early years to help develop secure, or repair insecure, attachments. In the absence of therapeutic or other professional specialized help, the following problematical aspects associated with attachment disorder might usefully be considered with activities to support them:

- A child overly concerned with attachment needs often depends too much on others for approval and self-validation. Activities aimed at finding a sense of self-worth can help with long-lasting, trusting relationships (e.g. 'Lack of self-esteem/confidence: My Hero', pp.96–102 and 'Abuse: The Shield', pp.42–48).

- A child who is fearful can be helped to learn to trust others which, in turn, may encourage him to invest in long-lasting, honest and mutually beneficial relationships.

- A child who refuses to be helped and is overly self-reliant can be encouraged to accept help from others by learning that rejection is not always the reaction to a request.

- Time spent looking at the subject of separations and reunions may help a child begin to consider these as a normal part of life rather than something to be dreaded or overly desired.

Trust activities

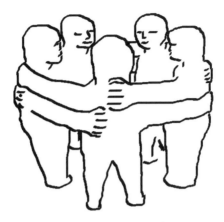

The following exercises explore the building of trust through bodywork and eye contact. Children for whom touch has not necessarily been a pleasant experience will normally take a while to trust the contact of others.

Note of caution: To comply with current legislation it is advised that all physical contact be between the children themselves with adults only directing the activities without becoming involved.

Application

These activities are best done with a small group of children, about six to ten. They are appropriate for very young children as well as ten- or eleven-year-olds. Children older than this who are becoming aware of their sexuality may be too embarrassed and the contact issues may need to be approached in another way.

Objectives

The aim of these activities is to encourage the child who is fearful to learn that it is possible to trust others, that physical contact does not necessarily involve pain or unpleasant feelings and that he is worthy of being 'seen'.

BACK TO BACK

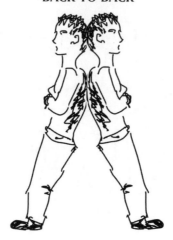

Resources
None

Application
It is easier to begin with this exercise since very shy children do not have to look each other in the face.

Exercise
- In pairs, ask the children to sit back to back.
- Ask them to say 'hello' through their backs to their partner.
- Divide each pair into an A and a B.
- Invite the A's to gently push their partner so that he has to lean forward.
- Swap to let B's have a turn.
- Invite both A's and B's to push simultaneously and see if they can raise their bottoms off the floor.
- See if any pair can actually stand up by pushing against their backs. (They may need to link arms to do this.)
- Discuss what happens when you push too much and how the best way is to feel and acknowledge each other's strength.

PUSH HANDS

Resources

None

Exercise

– Ask the children to face their partner and put the palms of their hands together.
– Pushing very gently on their palms, see if they can support each other while they move their feet apart.
– See how far apart they can move their feet, still supporting each other.
– Play with pushing partners through the hands to the point of nearly pushing them over and then stop.

GROUP FALL

Resources

Cushions or other soft landing material

Application

This exercise is more suitable for older children with enough strength to be able to support each other's weight.

Note of caution: Since this exercise has the potential for a child being allowed to fall, care should be taken that adequate cushioning is around and that the children concerned will take the exercise seriously.

Exercise

– Ask the children to stand in a tight circle with their shoulders touching. One child will be in the middle.
– Invite the child in the middle to imagine that he is weighted by his feet to the ground but can flop from side to side.
– As he flops, the children on that side will catch him, support him and gently return him to his feet.
– Encourage the child in the middle to really trust that he will be caught and give his whole weight to his supporters.
– If appropriate, discuss how it feels to be able to trust that others will support you when you need them.

JAILERS

Resources

Chairs (enough for half the number of children)

Application and objective

This exercise is aimed at encouraging children to be able to have open eye contact. This is best used before the '1, 2, 3' exercise (see below) since the element of fun helps minimize any anxiety.

> *Note of caution: Since children can become very excited playing this game, they should be cautioned not to grab each other by the neck or hair, etc.*

Exercise

- Place enough chairs for half the number of children in a circle. There should be one chair extra.
- Invite half the group to sit on the chairs and to be the 'prisoners'.
- Ask the rest of the group to take a chair and prisoner each and stand behind it as the 'jailers'. There should be one empty chair – one jailer without a prisoner.
- Make sure that the jailers are not standing too close to their prisoners (arm's length away is about right).
- The jailer who has no prisoner will wink (or blink for those who cannot wink) at one of the other prisoners who will then attempt to escape from his jailer and come to sit on the empty chair.
- After an appropriate time, the jailers and prisoners can swap over. (Someone will need to volunteer to play the jailer twice.)

1, 2, 3

Resources

None

Application

This is a group game, which can be played from about age six upwards to adult.

Objectives

The aim of this exercise is to encourage the children to seek out and maintain eye contact as well as be able to restrain from being diverted by others looking at them. Additionally the game helps children deal with the rejection of not having their 'look' or attention returned.

Exercise

- Ask the children to stand in a circle, a reasonable distance away from each other.
- Place an object in the centre of the circle and ask everyone to look at it.
- Together, everyone says 1, 2, and on the count of 3 looks towards another member of the group.
- If any two people happen to be looking at each other they can change places.
- Encourage the children not to cheat and look round to see who is looking at them.
- Praise any child you can see who avoids doing this but continues to look in the direction of someone who is not looking at him.
- If appropriate, discuss how it feels to have someone looking at you and not be able to return the attention. Also and more importantly discuss how it feels to be looking at someone and not have your attention returned.
- Again, if appropriate, this may lead to discussions of how rejection is not always actual or intended but may only be circumstantial or implied.

Further activities

Suggestions for books that provide further games and activities on trust are offered in Appendix 3.

Other issues addressed

All issues.

BEREAVEMENT
The issue

More and more children in our schools are suffering from a sense of loss, as parental separation in our society seems to be on the increase. Although it entails similar stages of grief, the issue of parental separation involves other complications and is dealt with later. When a child loses a grandparent, beloved pet or even a parent, sad though it is for him, if there are no traumatic circumstances surrounding the death, he will experience what is termed as *simple grief* and, to a greater or lesser extent, he will go through the normal stages of grieving in correlation with his emotional age. (Both the stages of grieving and the way children grieve will be explained in this section.) However, if there are other complicated issues surrounding the death of this significant person, then the experience for the child will be one of *complicated grief.*

It goes without saying that the issue of complicated grief is far more difficult to manage than that of simple grief where the stages basically run through shock and disbelief, denial, anger, acceptance, assimilation and moving on. (Complicated grief may need the support of a professional trained in this area.) There may be periods when one or other of these stages is revisited or when it feels that the child is experiencing more than one. In principle, however, there should only be cause for concern if a child seems to be stuck in one of these stages without any signs of progression.

The behaviours

Perhaps the most important point to remember is that *the way children grieve will, more often than not, be how their parents or carers grieve.* A recently widowed father may, for example, bring his child to me worried that the child does not want to talk about his mum. With gentle questioning I find out there are no photos of her in the house and that dad has taken on extra shifts to 'keep himself busy'.

Grief is personal and the way children grieve will be affected by many different circumstances: their character, environment, people around them, etc. The following is, therefore, only a generalization of the behaviours often found during the different stages of simple grief.

Shock and disbelief

The first stage of grief is normally that of shock or disbelief and may even be felt as physical pain or numbness. This is when the bereaved person catches glimpses of the deceased in a crowded street. Young children often upset their surviving parent by continually asking 'When is daddy/ mummy coming home?' Sometimes this stage is accompanied by what may seem unnatural calmness and it may be disconcerting for staff at school to see a child whose loved one has just died playing happily in the playground. It may be useful here to remember the adage: *children grieve in puddles.* That is to say, one minute they may be inconsolable and the next they are laughing at a cartoon on television. This is perfectly normal and the trick is to follow their lead. Make time to console and comfort them sufficiently and then distract them.

Denial

Here adults and older children may pretend they don't care and that everything is 'fine'. Hyperactivity often accompanies this stage as in the case of the dad working double shifts. A younger child may complain of a 'bad tummy' or headaches and if very young may become anxious on separation. If one person disappeared, then maybe another will! Insomnia may develop and little ones may regress to wetting the bed or refusing to sleep in their own rooms. Continual reassurance is needed that the world is still a safe place.

Anger

This stage revolves around a growing awareness that the loved person is not coming back. There may be a mixture of emotions but anger is usually one of them. It is important to reassure the child that it is perfectly okay to be angry and find ways to help him express his feelings. Children may use behaviour that is extreme in order to match the savagery of their emotions (see 'Anger', pp.48–54). Any or all of the following may be present: yearning or pining, anger at anyone or anything remotely connected to the death, desperate need to find reasons, feelings of emptiness and depression accompanied by lowered self-confidence and self-esteem. Guilt may be another emotion felt here, a typical example being that a child may feel if they had acted differently mummy or daddy might still be here, as in the case of the young girl who thought it her fault that her daddy had died of a heart attack (see 'A child's concept of reality', pp.29–31).

It is important here to get to the bottom of whatever is worrying the child and reassure him that it was not his fault. The issue may be trivial in our eyes, for example, not keeping a room tidy or feeding the cat, and it is sometimes hard for an adult to believe that a child could even entertain such an absurd notion. However, in my experience, they can and frequently do (see 'Parental separation', pp.115–122).

Acceptance, assimilation and moving on

Eventually, and there is no rule as to when this may happen, there is a certain acceptance of the death and an ability to begin to envisage life without the loved one. Significant times of celebration, that is, birthdays, anniversaries, Christmas, etc. play a particular role in the moving-on process in that the first year each of these is experienced without the deceased can be a traumatic and painful occasion. However, providing each occasion is invested with due ceremony and made special in its own right, the following years are normally less upsetting since memories of experiences without the loved one have already begun.

Assimilation is the final stage in bereavement and may never happen. The bereaved adult or child may simply form an acceptance of a kind with which they can live and start to move on in their own way. Assimilation comes when a true recognition of the deceased's life and legacy is integrated into the psyche of the bereaved so that they feel they have grown from having known their loved one.

Specific age-related behaviour

The above is a description of behaviours one might expect in general from adults as well as children but it might be useful to offer a brief explanation of specific age-related behaviour and the belief system that underpins it.

It is a common misconception that babies under the age of two do not grieve. Research has shown that very young children can and do become depressed. Their way of showing this is often by refusing to eat or sleep; they may cry incessantly or become very irritable. They may also become withdrawn and lose interest in their toys or, if they are mobile, constantly search for the missing person.

Between the ages of two and five a child will still not understand what death means since this an abstract concept (see 'Metaphor and symbol', pp.32–33). It is important not to use euphemisms such as 'Daddy's gone to sleep' or 'Mummy has gone on a long journey' since the child may well become terrified of going to sleep or on a journey himself. Simple, plain language is best, using concrete images such as dead birds or other symbols from nature. Fear of abandonment is strong and the child may begin to push boundaries to reassure himself that his world is still safe and there is still someone there who cares. (This behaviour does not only belong to this age group but may persist into adolescent years.) This is a disturbing stage for those managing bereaved children since a fine balance has to be struck between compassion for the child's grief and firm boundaries on his behaviour. It is tempting to excuse a bereaved child any misdemeanour but it is more comforting for him to know that he is still part of a loving, caring world that has the same boundaries and is continuing as normal.

By the time a child is eight he normally has some idea of what death means. At this age he is becoming aware of wider social structures and the implications this death may have on his close and wider family networks. This is where the issue of guilt, as previously discussed, may arise. More than ever a child of this age will need consistent and firm boundaries since he may regress to behaviour reminiscent of the more emotionally volatile pre-school child, including temper tantrums.

As a child grows older he becomes more aware of the totality and universality of death. In adolescence the issue is complicated by the teenager's hormonal changes and resultant rapid physical and emotional development. A trusted person who can support the adolescent in compartmentalizing his feelings is of great benefit here.

Objectives

When working with a bereaved child it may be useful to remember the following objectives for the activities:

- To make the loss real for the child, especially if there is a family culture of hiding facts and feelings. (This must obviously be done sensitively through working with the family as well.)

- To support the child through the period of change or transition (see 'Change or transition', pp.83–87).

- To help the child identify and express the sometimes very confusing emotions.

- To gently dispel any negative beliefs, for example, reason for death, attributed blame, etc.

- To help the child move on in his own time and form positive hopes for the future.

- If appropriate, to help the child see what he has gained from his relationship with the deceased.

Areas for concern

With patience, honesty and gentle but firm handling, most children can be guided through the process of simple grief. However, if a child appears to be stuck in one of the previously mentioned stages, or becomes unnaturally aggressive or withdrawn, then professional support should be sought. Similarly, if the death was violent or the circumstances surrounding it confusing or highly emotionally charged, then the child may be suffering from complicated grief or even PTSD (post-traumatic stress disorder).

This may be suspected if one or more of the following behaviours are present, in which case the child should be referred to a professional trained in this area:

- Repetitive play in which the themes or aspects of the death are expressed.

- Highly disorganized and/or frightened behaviour.

- Repeated flashbacks, either auditory or visual, of the event.

- Distressing and repetitive dreams of the event or frequent highly disturbing dreams without recognizable content.

Activities

YOU MAY THINK THIS IS A PIECE OF MATERIAL...

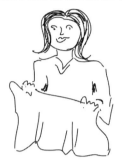

Resources

Brightly coloured material, at least a metre in width and length

Application

This exercise is best used with a group of children. Even very young children can be helped to use the mime and often come up with some good ideas of their own!

Objectives

This is a useful warm-up to the next activity, especially for some children who do not possess the kind of imagination that can see a piece of material as anything other than a piece of material!

It is important to preface each turn with the suggested words. This is for two reasons: first, the words endow the action with a sense of magic to make more believable the transformation of the material, and second, it introduces the act of ritual that puts a comforting structure around potentially emotional situations (see 'Change or transition', pp.83–87).

Exercise

– Tell the children you are going to play a guessing game with a piece of material.
– Say the first one who guesses correctly can have the next go.
– Pick up the material and say 'You may think this is a piece of material but actually it is a...'
– Pretend to vacuum the carpet with it. (You can obviously choose something else but this is an easy first choice.)
– Explain that every player must start his go with the words 'You may think...'

If the children need encouragement, televisions, dog leads, teapots or even parachutes and flying carpets make recognizable objects. Most children seem to take to this game and the suggestions can become quite creative and imaginative.

THE DRAGON STORY

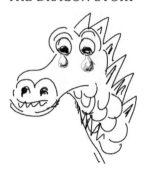

Resources
Multiple lengths of coloured material – blue, green, brown and black
Length of wallpaper
Felt tip pens or paints

Application and objective
This exercise can be done with an individual child but is more useful if performed with a group since the aim is to introduce this often-taboo subject so that the children can express their ideas, opinions and feelings through the safety of the story. The objective is to begin to normalize the idea of death and for the child in question to feel he is not alone in his grief. By physically moving the material and taking turns the children become part of the story and identify more strongly with it without the complications that might ensue from taking on a role. If there are specific issues that need to be addressed, then the story can be altered accordingly.

Exercise
- Seat the children in a wide circle and pile the material to one side of the middle.
- Explain you are gong to tell them a story with the material and they might like to finish it for you.
- Tell the following story or some derivation thereof, choosing a separate piece of material for each character or geographical aspect. Build up the picture on the floor.

Story suggestion

Once upon a time there was a country with many green fields [spread out green material] and many mountains [put more green material in two piles on either side]. Between the mountains there ran a deep blue river [length of blue material between green piles] and beside the river there was a village [brown material beside blue]. In one of the mountains, in a big cave lived Mr. and Mrs. Dragon [two different coloured pieces of material in one of the green piles such as pink and grey]. Mr. and Mrs. Dragon were very happy living there in their mountain. They did not speak to the village people and the village people did not speak to them. In fact, if any of the village people ventured up the mountain, Mr. Dragon would roar and breathe fire at them. [Use red material to mime this.] Then one day, something very sad happened. Mrs. Dragon died. Mr. Dragon cried and cried and then he buried Mrs. Dragon in another cave halfway up the mountain so that he could go and visit her at any time. [Bury pink material in green.] Time passed and Mr. Dragon was very lonely in his cave high up on the mountain all by himself. He often looked down and saw the village people [mime this] but he could not bring himself to go down. 'I don't need them,' he said to himself. 'I'm all right here by myself.' But he wasn't really; he was very, very lonely and would have loved to see a friendly face. In their turn the village people looked up at the mountain [mime this] and said, 'Should we go and see if he is all right?', but then they said, 'Oh no! He will only roar and breath fire at us and frighten us.' So they stayed in their village and Mr. Dragon stayed in his mountain.

Then one day something very unexpected happened. [You can end the story here or continue with the following:] The winds started to blow, a big, black storm arrived and it grew bigger and bigger and bigger. [Flap black material over the scene.]

- Now ask the children what they think happened next. Encourage them to take turns and move the material around or use fresh pieces to introduce new characters, objects or landscapes.

Note of caution: This story addresses the stage of denial and the all too frequent way bereaved people become introverted. It also addresses the confusion for others in knowing how to behave around a bereaved person. Although the group leader will have this in mind it is important to allow the children to make up their stories and to trust in the power of the metaphor (see 'Metaphor and symbol', pp.32–33) rather than directing the story oneself. The focus here is on the work being non-directive to allow the natural flow of self-healing to take place (see 'Directive and non-directive intervention', p.34), although issues of unacceptable behaviour will obviously need to be addressed. The story can be altered accordingly to address other topics such as anger or guilt.

Extensions

Once the children have completed their story, it can be drawn or painted on a roll of wallpaper as a frieze. This may be done in detail, or with younger children, just the colours to represent the characters, etc., with the odd word may suffice.

Further activities

- The seasons of nature offer a good source of material for dealing with the cycles of birth, life, death and rebirth. Drama activities can include a series of group sculpts (see 'Using drama techniques', pp.35–37) with the children being seeds, full-grown plants or trees, bearing fruit, withering, withdrawing and dying only to start again from seed. The emphasis here is on normalizing death and helping the child to understand it is an integral and important part of life.

- Embodying or using body sculpts (see 'Using drama techniques', pp.35–37) of any of the feelings that may be present such as sadness, anger, guilt, anxiety, betrayal, rejection, helplessness, loneliness, panic, shame, depression, restlessness, weariness, emptiness, relief, gladness and freedom.

- There are many other activities suitable for supporting bereaved children such as making memory boxes, writing a letter to the special person, making salt sculptures (colouring salt with chalks and layering in a glass jar to represent the different attributes of the deceased). As a general rule an art or craft activity is more appropriate *after* a drama exercise as it makes more concrete those feelings evoked by the drama.

Other issues addressed

Anger and change or transition.

BULLYING

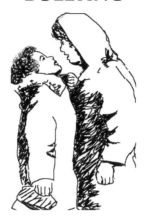

The issue

Bullying has now, fortunately, become recognized as an issue in most schools to the extent that most schools have an anti-bullying policy, which should be available for all parents to see. Obviously, schools differ in their approach to bullying from the 'we don't have any bullying in our school' attitude, which often means the bullying is ignored, to the 'we do not tolerate bullies', which is generally more effective. Anti-bullying strategies are often linked to school councils or PSHE (Personal Social Health and Economic education).

Bullying can take many forms ranging from physical harm to name-calling. It can be verbal, emotional, physical or, less commonly, sexual. Most often it is a combination of verbal and emotional, with children 'picking on' others with racist, homophobic or just generally abusive remarks.

Very often it will be one particular characteristic about a child that will make them vulnerable. It may be appearance, disability, race, family circumstances, sexual orientation or merely body language. This last plays an important part in whether a child is going to be bullied, whatever other handicap he may have, and measures can be taken to help a child in this way. A more recent form of bullying is cyber bullying when a child receives *persistent*, inappropriate and often abusive texts and photos online or through their mobile phone.

The key concept in all bullying is the word *persistent* since a one-off, hurtful comment or act may stem from other mitigating circumstances. Persistence implies determination and a resolution to achieve one's goal; it cannot be attributed to a 'mistake' or something someone did not 'mean' to do, excuses often used by bullies.

Although the idea of bullying usually conjures up images of a bigger child intimidating a smaller child, a more insidious and less manageable form is that which is not overt but goes unseen and unnoticed by school staff. This is the bullying by omission: the not talking to someone, deliberately and *persistently* leaving them out of a game, organizing or intimidating other children to do the same. The victim of this kind of bullying may simply become more and more withdrawn, but the process can be so slow that it may be difficult for staff to spot until the child becomes school phobic or chronically depressed.

A fact that is commonly known but is often, understandably, overlooked in the heat of the moment is that a bully is usually being, or has been, bullied. By exerting his power and control, whether by force or omission, he is simply trying to regain that sense of self-esteem, self-confidence or identity, which has been taken away from him. In energy terms he is trying to fill the void inside himself by feeding off another. Whether from jealousy, a need to be the centre of attention, a need for power and control, bullying nearly always stems from a lack of self-confidence because the bully has never been praised or made to feel good at home. Using threatening tactics will therefore only serve to diminish that lack of self-worth that the bully already feels and, in many cases, perpetuate a script with which he is already familiar.

The behaviours

The spectrum of presenting behaviours pertaining to bullying is as wide as the many forms it takes. These behaviours may range from slight introversion on the part of the child being bullied to attempted or actual suicide. There are many online help organizations that offer support to children and parents and give extensive information on what behaviours to look out for (see Appendix 3). The following is a list compiled from this information:

- Bed wetting, nightmares or being unable or unwilling to go to sleep when there has been no previous history of such.

- Suddenly wanting a lift to school rather than taking the bus, changing the route to school, finding excuses not to go to school, for example, feigning illness, or truanting from school.

- A deterioration in grades or marks at school where before the child was achieving well.

- Acquiring nervous habits: hair pulling, skin scratching, nervous tics or stammers.

- Avoiding certain people or activities.

- Starting to bully others, either other children at school or younger siblings. The child is possibly modelling his bullying behaviour on that of another member of the family.

- Coming home regularly with clothes or books destroyed or very hungry, which might signify that lunch money, or lunch itself, has been taken.

- Beginning to steal or ask for money to pay the bully.

- Becoming uncharacteristically aggressive or unreasonable.

- Losing appetite for food or refusing to eat.

- Attempting or threatening suicide.

- Refusing to talk or giving improbable or impossible reasons for any of the above.

Areas for concern

Although most issues of bullying can be quickly and reasonably resolved, especially if detected early, there appear to be an ever increasing number of incidents where children have found the only alternative to living with bullying is to take their own lives. If a child is self-harming or threatens suicide, that is, *if he is at risk of significantly harming himself or others*, then referral to the appropriate professionals should be made via the head or principal of the school *without delay*.

Activities

THE STATUS GAME/I'M OK

Resources
None

Application
As previously mentioned body language can play an enormous part in whether or not a child is going to be bullied. The following exercise can be

used on an individual basis, but (since bullying often involves more than one person) is possibly more effective with a group when positive feedback from peers can be given.

Objective

To encourage the child to use body language which does not immediately make him a target for bullies.

Exercise

- Explain to the children that there are ways in which they can help to protect themselves from being bullied.
- Tell the children that if they have 'I am a victim' or 'I am open to being bullied' written all over them, then they probably will be.
- Say that you are going to experiment with how to say 'I am not a victim' and 'I am not going to be bullied' through the language of their bodies so that they are protected. (You might like to preface this exercise with 'In the Mirror', p.80.)
- Explain that the trick is about staying calm and saying little or even nothing at all, letting your body do the talking.
- Invite one child to go to a corner of the room and tell him that he is going to play the part of the bully.
- Invite another child to go to the opposite corner and tell him that he has 'I am going to be bullied' written all over him. Discuss with the group how this looks.
- Ask the children to move slowly towards each other and stop when they are opposite each other.
- Enquire as to how each child is feeling and discuss with the group how easy it might be for the bullying to take place.
- Using the same two children (so that the previous 'victim' is not left feeling depleted) ask the bully to remain in character while the victim changes his body language to 'I am not a victim' and 'I am not going to be bullied'. Again, discuss with the group how this looks.
- Ask the children to move towards each other as before and stop when together.
- Enquire as to whether their feelings towards each other have changed. Does the bully feel as confident about bullying now?
- Allow different members of the group to have a go at being the victim and practise walking calmly and confidently across the room, standing their ground when face-to-face with the bully.

– Remember to *derole* the children (see 'Using drama techniques', pp.35–37) so that they do not carry the character back into the classroom.

Extensions

Depending on the age and cognitive ability of the children this activity can be extended into a piece of improvisation/drama work as follows:

- Allow the victim, on meeting the bully, to slowly come out of his victim body language and change to the more confident stance. See if this changes the body language of the bully.

- Practise moving slightly away from the bully and repeating one or two specific phrases (as in 'A Broken Record'; see 'Lack of self-esteem/confidence', pp.96–102). These need to be neutral and cheerful such as 'See you later' or 'No thanks, not this time'. Known as *denial skills*, these derive from a martial arts technique, which has as its subtext 'Don't be there'.

- With older children this exercise can be extended into a piece of drama that involves *reframing* (see 'Parental separation', pp.115–122 and 'Using drama techniques', pp.35–37), when the altered body language and denial skills can change the outcome of the confrontation.

Further activities

In schools that include work on body language as part of their curriculum, this next activity may not be necessary. However, it may serve as a useful reminder as to the importance of our body image and the messages we are giving to others.

IN THE MIRROR

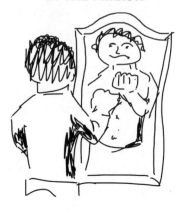

Resources
None

Application
This activity can be done with the use of an actual mirror or by *mirroring* the child's body posture yourself (see 'Using drama techniques', pp.35–37).

Objectives
This exercise is usefil as a way of encouraging a child to understand how his feelings can translate into body language and how other people may relate either positively or negatively to this.

Exercise
- Using a full-length mirror ask the child to pretend to think of something really sad and then look at himself in the mirror.
- Then ask him to think of something really happy and look again.
- Discuss what you both see and ask him to make the 'sad' gesture bigger (head more drooped, shoulders more hunched, etc.).
- Do the same for the 'happy' feeling.
- Ask him to go slowly from one exaggerated posture to the other and discuss what is happening in his body and how each makes him feel.
- Ask him what he would think about someone he met who looked like this.
- Think of some positive statements he could say, for example, 'I will find someone else to play with' to replace any hurtful words and practise this when in the 'happy' posture.

'I NEED YOU TO LISTEN'

Resources
None

Application
Sometimes a child may not, for a variety of reasons, be listened to or heard when complaining about being bullied. Using drama to help a child stand up for himself and get his needs met can be very effective. A useful technique here is *role reversal* (see 'Using drama techniques', pp.35–37) since, through mirroring, it allows the child to see himself as he appears to the adult. If handled in a light-hearted way this exercise can be fun and can produce much laughter that, in turn, helps the child to relax.

Objectives
The objective here is to encourage the child to be confident enough to state his needs calmly when in a stressful situation.

Exercise
-   Rehearse with the child what he might say to a teacher or parent if he is being bullied. As the adult pretend that you are too busy or too tired to listen to him.
-   Swap roles and repeat the scenario, mirroring the approach that the child has just taken. (This should be done carefully so that the child does not feel demeaned in anyway.)
-   Ask the child (in his role as adult) what you (as the child) would need to do to make him listen to you.
-   Follow his instructions. Hopefully he will make suggestions like 'Stand up taller', 'Speak more loudly', etc. If not, you may have to make these suggestions yourself.
-   Reverse roles again and allow the child, as himself, to rehearse the different approach.
-   It is also worth practising the 'A Broken Record' technique (see 'Lack of self-esteem/confidence', pp.96–102) to encourage the child to be persistent in stating their needs. Phrases such as 'I really need you to listen to me' and 'I'm feeling really bad about this' if continually and calmly stated should produce the desired results.

CHANGING THE PLAY

Resources

None

Application

The background to this activity is explained in 'Using drama techniques: Reframing' (pp.35–37) and is interchangeable with the 'Reframing/Trying Again' activity in 'Parental separation' (pp.115–122). In this context it can be a very useful tool to explore with groups the emotional impact and possible alternative outcomes to a situation involving bullying. Because it involves role-playing and improvisation, the majority of children under the age of about nine will find it difficult to engage with this activity. In my experience it works best with teenagers, especially if they have had some drama teaching.

Objectives

The objective is to explore scenarios where bullying may be prevented by something someone says, does or even just by their body language.

Note of caution: Since this exercise involves the use of extended drama it is advised that some training in drama skills be undertaken first.

Exercise

- Discuss with the group possible scenarios in which bullying might occur and make a list of these on the board or a flip chart.
- Use one or more of the warm-up games (see 'Group warm-up games', pp.40–41).
- Divide the class into groups of at least three (depending on their drama abilities: the more in a group, the more difficult the role-play).
- Ask each group to choose and improvise a different scenario. (*Freeze frames* (see 'Using drama techniques, pp.35–37) can be used here if the groups have difficulty getting straight into role-play.)
- Once the groups have rehearsed, allow each group to present their work to the others.
- Once all groups have presented their work and been duly congratulated on it, explain that you are going to take one of the scenarios and look at how an alternative (and more positive) outcome might occur if one of the actors at some stage said or did something differently. Discuss how this might come about, that is, an action, repeated phrase, body language or combination of all of these.

- Ask one of the groups to play through their scenario again and explain to the others that they are to watch very carefully to find the trigger point at which they feel events could be changed.

- At this point any of the spectators can shout 'Stop' and either take the place of that particular actor to change the turn of events, or tell the actor what he could do differently. (Which of these two techniques is used will depend on the temperaments of the young people involved, that is, whether the actor objects to having to stand down.)

- Make sure the technique of *deroling* (see 'Using drama techniques', pp.35–37) is employed fully to ensure no one carries the emotions of their role back into class.

Note of caution: Although this activity can be conducted safely, we are dealing here with heightened emotions and care should be taken to derole the actors and choose a suitable calming exercise to finish with (see 'Closure activities', pp.143–145). In addition, it is not advisable to allow a child who has been seriously bullied to play that part in the enactment in case he becomes re-traumatized. This activity can be used with other issues (see 'Other issues addressed', below) but the same proviso will hold, that a child who has been seriously affected by the situation should NOT replay the part of the victim.

Extensions

This form of activity obviously lends itself to group discussion before, during or after the role-play. With older children and/or those who are more emotionally literate, the technique of *speaking from role* (see 'Using drama techniques', pp.35–37) can be used to elicit a deeper understanding of motives.

Other issues addressed

Anxiety, change or transition, lack of self-esteem/confidence, learnt behaviour and socially inappropriate behaviour.

CHANGE OR TRANSITION

The issue

It is fairly obvious to most of us that some children cope better with change than others. Whereas my eldest child always took a disruption in her routine of catching the bus home in her stride, my youngest used to drive her teacher mad by asking every half an hour whether she was being picked up and was, as her primary school called it, a 'home child' rather than a 'bus child'. Two children from the same home, brought up in a similar way, with two entirely different reactions!

At any one time the changes facing children at school and home may be far greater than modes of transport. Simply moving from one class up into the next may provoke such feelings of terror in a sensitive child that he may invent illnesses or become a school refuser. These days, with parental separation on the increase, many children have to cope with moving from one house to another and from one primary carer to another as part of their weekly schedule, and their reaction to living in this constant state of uncertainty may manifest itself in a variety of disturbing behaviours. These behaviours may differ depending on the age of the child and, although a resilience to change may be acquired over time in some children, I would venture to suggest, from experience, that the feelings remain; it is only the degree and scope of the reaction that alters.

It is also well known that children on the autistic spectrum find coping with change more difficult than their peers. Changes that occur normally in the course of everyday school life may present as abnormal and frightening to a sensitive child or one who perceives the world differently. A change of classroom, an assembly at a different time or in a different place, a new teacher – any of these can disrupt a child's sense of safety and security to the extent that they will try to retreat from this scary new world, often by hiding under tables or finding other means, sometimes destructive, of remaining in control.

In addition to the already mentioned general issues involving change with which a child may be faced, there are, of course, the major times of transition which, on the whole, we do not acknowledge in our Western society today. Education is beginning to understand that events such as transition from pre-school to primary and primary to secondary school require extra input and primary/secondary liaison activities are the norm in many places. Outside school, however, life-changing occurrences such as a young boy's voice breaking or a young girl reaching puberty go largely unacknowledged. Drama and the use of ritualistic action can be enormously helpful to mark these times of transition, mirroring perhaps the way that major life changes were always dealt with in indigenous tribal societies.

The behaviours

Adults often underestimate the effect that change can have on some children. Faced with situations in which they feel out of control, children may resort to a variety of behaviours that attempt to put them back in control. These behaviours may range from hiding under tables to create their own manageable environment, to 'splitting' – creating an alter ego, which may be another person or an animal that (in the child's mind) copes better with the situation (see 'General and differentiated approaches', pp.28–29). The important issue is to remember that these behaviours are an attempt by the child to feel in control of an uncontrollable situation and that as adults we need either to change the situation or help the child feel more in control.

We can do this by putting structure around the child and activities that involve ritualistic action and repetition can help produce this supportive environment.

Activities

THE TWO ISLANDS

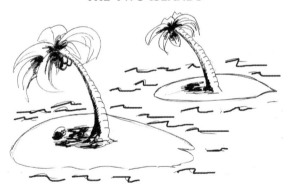

Resources
Lengths of coloured material

Application
This activity is useful when children are faced with an imminent major change in their lives of which they are aware, such as Year 6 transition to secondary school, a house move or even, for a more vulnerable child, progression into the next class.

Objective

The objective here is to use the metaphor of two islands to help the child understand and feel better about what is going to happen and to look at ways that will make the transition easier.

Exercise

- Make two different islands out of material (rugs or cushions can also be used).
- Allow the child to think carefully about the shape and colour of these islands as they represent the present and future.
- Ask the child to sit on the 'present' island and tell you how it feels to be there – the good and bad feelings about being in this class/house/school.
- Ask him then to look across at the 'future' island and tell you how he feels about having to go there. Try to elicit 'good and 'bad' feelings.
- When he is ready ask him if he would like to go across to this 'future' island and how he would like to go, for example, by stepping-stones, boat, plane, etc.
- Ask him if there is someone or something he would like to take with him from the 'present' island to help him with the transition.
- Allow the child time to move across to the island. If he refuses to go, ask him what would make it easier.
- Sit with the child on the 'future' island and ask him how he feels now.
- Ask the child how he feels looking back at what is now the 'past' island.

Extensions

The two islands can be used to represent any situations in the child's life that involve change, including people. Positive affirmations can be made about the new situation or island and used in repetition in a made-up poem or song. The islands can be drawn, depicted in a collage or sculpted in clay.

Further activities

As already mentioned, ritualistic action is very useful in providing a sense of safety and security for children, especially in times of change. We are using ritualistic action when we give out certificates and applaud in an assembly, and it is all the more effective when it is being witnessed by school, class or peer group. There are many ways this can be used within class time to empower a vulnerable child and increase his self-esteem and sense of security. The following are some ideas:

- Use the activity of 'The Two Islands' as a group, applauding as each child crosses over to the 'new' or 'future' island.

- Make 'shields' with the children (see 'Abuse', pp.42–48) and then present the shields by 'knighting' each child. The children stand in two lines and each child walks down the centre to kneel in front of the teacher who, with a makeshift sword, presents the shield and 'knights' the child as the class applauds.

- Tell the story of the 'Sword in the Stone', emphasizing how those who appear the strongest and cleverest are not always those who succeed best in life. There are other qualities, etc. Act out the pulling of the sword from the stone, allowing each child in turn to be Arthur. You may wish to run this activity after the last, with each child affirming his knighthood and/or qualities.

Other issues addressed

Bereavement, lack of self-esteem/confidence and parental separation.

COMPULSIVE LYING

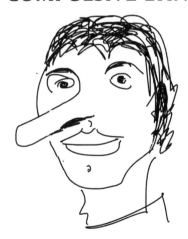

The issue

We have all met the child who appears to be a compulsive liar, who makes up stories at the drop of a hat, and who does not seem to know the difference between fact and fiction. This sort of child can pose huge problems for the teacher or adult in charge of the group or class, especially when the stories he tells involve worrying or potential safeguarding issues. In my work as a dramatherapist in inner-city schools I was asked to support a child who had been threatening to strangle another child with a scarf. When asked why, he replied that the voices of monsters in his head had told him to do it and that if he did not agree he would be killed. In the case of this particular child, he was partially telling the truth since there were, indeed, voices in his head in the form of soundtracks from horror films on a television left on all night by his sister who was scared of the dark. This boy's monsters had come directly from a particular film and he was convinced they were real.

This inability to distinguish between fact and fantasy is common in young children who, under a certain age, usually about seven, find abstract concepts very difficult (see 'Metaphor and symbol', pp.32–33). This is why it is difficult for a very young child to understand death (see 'Bereavement', pp.66–74) and why a child needs explanations that involve concrete realities in order to understand abstract ideas. When children are bombarded with films which contain fantastic characters, they have a tendency to believe in them which is all very well if the characters are fairies or talking teddy bears. When the characters are horrific and, more dangerously, when they increase their credibility by resembling humans, children under a certain age will not necessarily realize they are only products of the imagination.

Another reason why children may lie compulsively is to gain attention or to fabricate an ideal world that allows them to live out a fantasy. A child who is constantly blamed or criticized may also distort the truth to avoid punishment or to attract reward. Such children often grow up trying to please by saying what they think the adult wants them to say whether or not it bears any resemblance to the truth.

The behaviours

It is easy to become exasperated with a child who is constantly deceitful or tells barefaced lies but it is worthwhile remembering that there is always a reason why they are doing so.

If you are faced with a child who lies compulsively it may be helpful to ask yourself the following questions:

- What is the emotional age of this child and is it possible they are being exposed to unsuitable material? Are they merely confusing fact and fiction?

- Is the child creating a fantasy world to escape from an unacceptable reality?

- Is the child overly scared of punishment or are they very sensitive to criticism?

Note of caution: In any of the above cases it is, obviously, necessary to follow appropriate procedures and refer to the relevant child protection or safeguarding officer if there is any cause for concern. Once safeguarding issues have been dealt with, the following activity can help a child differentiate between fact and fantasy, truth and lies.

Activity

THE DIVIDED ROOM/FIBS AND FACT

Resources

Cushions
Lengths of coloured material
Puppets or small figures if necessary

Application

This activity can be used in any situation in which a child consistently tells lies, whether through misunderstanding, desire to please or avoidance of reality. In the latter two cases, repercussions of the lying can be explored either directly or through metaphor (see 'Further activities', below).

Note of caution: This exercise should not be used with children where there is known domestic violence at home. This should remain the province of the therapist.

Exercise

- Explain to the child that you are going to divide the room into half and that in one half you will both be able to tell stories that are not true, like fairy stories, and in the other you will talk about things that are true, such as how many pets you have, who you live with and what you had for dinner.

- Ask the child how they want to decorate the two halves of the room: for example, pink material and cushions may represent fairy stories (you may prefer to talk about fibs with an older child) while blue may be fact. Allow the child time to choose his materials and arrange the room since this is all part of the process.

- Sit with the child in the 'fact' half of the room and take it in turns to say one true statement each about yourself. With younger children try to stick to subjects which are concrete realities such as pets or people or colours of bedrooms, etc.

- Move across to the 'fairy tale' or 'fibs' half of the room, and either with or without the aid of small figures, soft toys or puppets, make up some stories.

- These made-up stories may include material from television or computer games, especially if the child is still worried or frightened by the characters. By firmly placing them in the 'fibs' half of the room, the child can be reassured that they pose no concrete threat.

- Continue this process over some weeks until the child can use the activity in the outside world and easily differentiate between reality and fantasy.

Extensions

Communication with other adults over the activity being used to help the child can help speed up the process. Usually the younger child comes to regard this activity as a game and is highly delighted that other adults are in the 'know' with regards whether something he has said comes from the 'blue, fact' or 'pink, fib' side of the room. With the older child or one who is consciously lying, turning the activity into a 'game' is obviously not appropriate, and a discussion or work on choices and consequences of actions may need to be undertaken (see 'Learnt behaviour: Consequences', pp.103–106).

Further activities

If a discussion on the consequences of lying is necessary, this can be done directly or may sometimes be more effective if done through metaphor (see 'Metaphor and symbol', pp.32–33). Fairy stories are a rich resource for archetypal 'good' and 'bad' qualities and can be read, or even better, acted out, with subsequent discussions on what the characters could have done differently. The technique of *reframing* (see 'Using drama techniques', pp.35–37) is useful here too.

- Pinocchio is an obvious choice for the subject of telling fibs.

Other issues addressed

Anxiety, lack of self-esteem/confidence and nightmares.

DEPRESSION

The issue

Many people suffer from feelings of sadness or, at times, hopelessness. Depression can be said to be present when these feelings persistently get in the way of normal activities. Even as late as the 1980s it used to be thought that only adults suffered from depression but now it is known that even small children and babies can be affected. According to the BBC Health website (2011), at least 2 per cent of children under the age of 12 have 'significant depression', which is to say that in a school of 300 there may be as many as 6 children suffering from depression at any one time.

Many factors can contribute to the causes of depression. These can be classed as reactive, for example, responses to circumstances such as parental divorce or separation or death of a loved one; they can be endogenous: that is to say, biological or genetic; or (a factor which is becoming increasingly prevalent nowadays) traumatic: a result of child abuse, conflict or emotional harm.

Factors that may produce depression in children may be one or a combination of the following:

- Divorce, separation or severe constant conflict of parents.
- Death or irretrievable loss of a loved one.
- Substantial change, for example, at home or school.
- Physical illness in self or primary carer.

- Ongoing pressure or stress, for example, at school or with exams.
- Feelings of rejection within the family or peer group.
- Extreme poverty or homelessness.

More than once during the course of my work I have come across children who may be said to operate permanently in the depressive mode. In simple terms they seem to 'care too much'. Overwhelmed by a sense of responsibility and often guilt and overly sensitive to the thoughts and feelings of others, they are quick to take the blame which, in turn, produces a lack of self-worth and confidence. They may appear mature beyond their age and adults around them are often lulled into a false sense of their emotional stability. Sometimes treated as emotional equals, these children, who seem to have the knack of picking up the slightest nuances of relationships and situations, will then take on the problems and worries of their elders. This in turn may render them incapable of living in the carefree and spontaneous world of the child and indulging in any activities involving make believe, imagination or the 'lighter' side of life.

This sort of child may become the emotional crux for a parent and may even 'download' his parent's problems to an extent where they manifest similar or even more severe symptoms or disturbances in behaviour.

The behaviours

Chronic low-level depression in children is very hard to identify and may go undiagnosed and treated for a long time, if not indefinitely. More identifiable depression may manifest itself in a variety of ways, including:

- Refusal to go to school or playing truant.
- Becoming very withdrawn, constantly moody, irritable or generally unhappy.
- Lack of concentration or interest in anything.
- Violent outbursts, disruptive behaviour, for example, bullying or stealing.
- Physical symptoms such as headaches, tummy aches, etc. whose causes remain unknown.
- Constant self-blame accompanied by lack of self-worth.

Specific age-related behaviour

Even babies and younger children may be able to pick up the moods of people around them and, coupled with an inability to understand what is going on, may manifest their feelings of sadness and hopelessness in refusal to eat, constant crying, irritability, clinginess, unresponsiveness or regression in development such as potty training or bed wetting.

With teenagers or older children, in addition to the behaviours mentioned above, there may be an addiction to drugs or alcohol or a lack of concern for one's own safety that manifests itself in a tendency to get into dangerous situations. Major changes in weight may press alarm bells or a predilection for horror movies or films, literature and websites that emphasize the 'darker' side of life. These children may also have a tendency to self-harm or may even overdose.

Supporting activities

If you are concerned about a child who may be exhibiting any of the above behaviours, the first response should obviously be to seek professional advice. The following are suggestions to support children with low-level depression or who are awaiting clinical assessment:

- Discuss with the child short-term achievable tasks and goals and support him to follow through with these.

- If possible encourage the child to take part in extra-curricular activities, particularly those that involve physical exercise, since research shows that this has a beneficial effect on pathways in the brain.

- Offer encouragement to talk but do not react if the offer is refused.

- Listen if they want to talk, but do not insist.

- Show that you believe what they say.

- Respect any defences the child may have.

- Some children may respond to the symbolism of myths and stories that extend the imagination but also deal with the more serious side of life.

Activities

OPPOSITE CORNERS

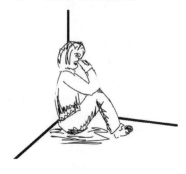

Resources

None

Application

This exercise can be used with one or more children.

Objectives

The objectives of this and the following exercises are to encourage the child to identify and acknowledge his different feelings. Those trapped in depression have described it as the lack of ability to distinguish between shades of black and white emotion, everything seeming to appear on a continuum of hopeless grey. The aim is therefore to help the child to separate out and compartmentalize his feelings so that the whole does not appear to be more than the sum of its parts.

Exercise

- With the child think of two 'big, bad feelings', for example, angry, sad or frightened.
- Again, together think of what their opposites might be, for example, calm, happy, comforted.
- Draw these feelings in any way the child wishes on four separate sheets of paper and put in four separate corners of the room, opposite feelings on the diagonal.
- With the child think of some situations which can apply to anyone, for example, Christmas, a birthday, being told off by a teacher, being bullied, and ask him to place himself somewhere on the line between the opposite emotions. For example, he may be very near the happy

drawing for Christmas and birthday and near the angry or frightened drawing for being told off or bullied.

- Having spent a while playing with these 'general' events, suggest you take it in turns to think of things that have specifically happened to you and place yourself at the appropriate place.
- This could be turned into a guessing game if appropriate.

Extensions

As a way of encouraging 'embodiment' of different feelings (see 'Underpinnings of dramatherapy', pp.32–34) play with how you would show each other what 'a little bit happy/sad/angry/frightened', etc. might look like as opposed to 'a lot' by moving from one corner to the other.

Further activities

Since symbolism often appeals to children who suffer from depression, the following activities may be useful:

- With older children a lifeline can be drawn using the metaphor of a river or a journey over mountains, etc. to show the ups and downs of their lives so far.

- Working with clay is a comforting displacement activity and a child may be encouraged to mould an animal or bird and tell a story about it which should remain in the metaphor (see 'Underpinnings of dramatherapy', pp.32–34).

- In an effort to explain to a child how everything sometimes seems so jumbled up that the mess appears hopeless, I often use the analogy of a chest of drawers, the contents of which have been emptied out onto the floor. Children often enjoy drawing this mess while I draw the chest with its empty drawers. The child can then be encouraged to put (draw) some items back into the drawers.

Note of caution: Especially with younger children this exercise should also remain in the metaphor unless the child specifically wants to talk about it.

Other issues addressed

Anger, anxiety, bereavement, bullying, change or transition, lack of self-esteem/confidence and parental separation.

LACK OF SELF-ESTEEM/CONFIDENCE
The issue

There may be many reasons why a child may suffer from a lack of self-esteem, confidence or, at the top end of the scale, a lack of a sense of his own identity. These may, for example, be inherited genetic traits; place in the family; multiple changes in the family or home; loss; bereavement; neglect; abuse; parental expectations; over-critical, absent or inconsistent parenting.

Many children are termed 'shy' and no one would wish for a class of extraverts! On the whole I, personally, would only regard this 'shyness' as a problem if it is inhibiting a child from achieving his full potential or he is clearly suffering because of it. Lack of a sense of one's own identity, that is, not really knowing who you are, especially in relation to others, is, however, an entirely different matter and much more serious, often necessitating a professional therapeutic intervention.

Very low self-esteem may stem from a lack of love in early childhood. Research has shown that certain chemicals in the brain (oproids and oxytocin among others), responsible for helping us feel good about ourselves, are released when a child is in a constantly warm, loving and unconditional relationship (Sunderland 2006). Lack of love may mean a child could grow up with an absence of these chemicals in the brain and self-doubt will be compounded by the deepening of the neural pathways in the brain that channel negative thoughts.

I have met children whose opinion of themselves is so low that they cannot bear to be praised, regarding it as a totally alien and unacceptable script, so different from the one they know. These are the often difficult-to-reach children, and work through projective play may need to be done to distance the situation and soften the emotional impact (see 'Underpinnings of dramatherapy', pp.32–34).

If a child has experienced trauma or neglect in early childhood then he may find it difficult to form a healthy concept of himself as apart and different from others. Dr. Peter Levine, a world authority on healing trauma, tells us that cruelty and neglect inflicted on children at strategic developmental stages in their lives can result in symptoms that resemble the trauma of shock (see 'Trauma and shock', pp.139–141). He goes on to say that children who have experienced developmental trauma should be referred to a therapist to help them work through the issues that are connected with their traumatic reactions (Levine 1997).

This is the top end of the scale where professional help should be sought, but there are many children out there who have experienced the 'small shocks' of everyday difficult family living and/or inadequate parenting and whose self-esteem has taken a battering. These children may benefit from drama exercises, which allow them to experience themselves as something or someone special so that their role repertoire (see 'Underpinnings of dramatherapy', pp.32–34) is extended and they begin to see different ways of relating to others.

Consistent cruelty and neglect can have an equally detrimental effect on a child's ability to see himself as others or to be able to put himself in another's shoes – another strategic developmental phase. This child may be lacking in empathy since he has retreated into himself and created his own safe world inside. Severe manifestations of this sort of behaviour should obviously be treated by a qualified therapist, but a child who simply finds it difficult to relate to others, or to understand how others feel, may benefit from rehearsing social situations either in role or using the projective medium of puppets or small figures.

The behaviours

Fear of the loss of a parent's love can have devastating effects on a child. If a child's demand for, or offer of, affection is met with indifference, withdrawal or other inappropriate response, then a 'fight or flight' reaction can be triggered in the lower brain. A 'fight' reaction will result in anger or aggression and a 'flight' response in depression or social withdrawal.

It is, of course, not always appropriate to blame the parents in this scenario since there may be many reasons why they may find it difficult to respond to their child in a suitably loving way. Most often, in my experience, it is because they themselves have received inadequate parenting and simply do not know how to deal with their fretful, demanding offspring.

Sometimes, as a result of illness or trauma, they have retreated into an emotional unresponsiveness to the world in general and cannot bring themselves to react with the joyful and loving spontaneity, which triggers the 'feel-good' chemicals and hormones in their child's brain. This was so with a child referred to me and assessed by the mental health team as having two years delay in emotional development. Her mother, as a result of consistent domestic abuse, had withdrawn emotionally from life. Her child had her needs met in every way except emotionally, graphically and poignantly outlined through the metaphor of her story of a puppy whose mummy could not help her because a big, big elephant was sitting on her.

Equally, a child may eventually respond with hatred: hatred of himself and the world in general. If, when little, he has learnt that his reaching out to his parent only meets with negativity, he may then come to the conclusion that he does not deserve this love, that there must be something wrong with him and that it is all his fault. By using hateful, negative behaviour, he can be assured of at least *some* sort of reaction, which is possibly more than he was getting originally.

A child may also respond by incessantly trying to please the adults around him as if, by doing so, he can earn the love that he is being denied.

Areas for concern

It has already been advised that presenting behaviours that include alarming reactions, such as actual or threatened harm to oneself or others, should be referred without delay to a mental health team. Furthermore, if a child continues to be inexplicably withdrawn despite all efforts to engage him, then he will also need the support of a professional trained in this area.

Activities

MY HERO

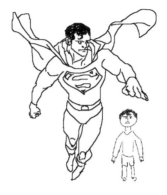

Resources

Lengths of coloured material
Masks (optional)
Dressing-up clothes (optional)

Application

I have used this technique on numerous occasions with some good results in terms of self-empowerment for the child. It is most effective if used on an individual basis with the adult playing all the additional characters (an often daunting task!). A non-therapist can use it safely, providing certain considerations are taken into account as follows:

- After the initial set-up, let the child lead the enactment. He should be the director in all cases unless he appears to be rehearsing violent, cruel or otherwise inappropriate behaviour, in which case the effect on the recipient should be pointed out and the enactment diverted into a more suitable scenario.

- It is especially important for the adult not to give her own ideas since we may be dealing here with children who have a tendency to try to please. Following the child's lead and reaffirming his ideas or actions will help him establish a sense of his own importance.

Objectives

The objective is to encourage the child to find within himself those qualities which will build his resilience. Externalizing and personifying these qualities make it easier for him to recognize and acknowledge them as his own.

Exercise

- Ask the child to tell you who is his hero. If possible this should not be a real life person since this may well be a footballer and thus limit the enactment to kicking a ball!

- If the child needs further prompting, discuss his favourite film, TV programme or book. Avoid anything that contains gratuitous violence. If in doubt ask the child about his favourite fairy story.

- Suggest that you play out some scenes from the film/book/TV programme, with the child playing his favourite character. Say you will be everyone else!

- Set the scene by using material to transform the room, for example, blue for the sea, green for the mountains, etc. (Quite a bit of imagination is needed here, but most children find this much easier than adults.)

- Invite the child to choose material, a costume or mask to transform himself into the character.

- Talk about the scenes you are going to enact. You may suggest your play has a beginning, middle and an end, but do not worry if it is far less structured than that. The child will be playing through what he needs to.

- Follow the child's lead and 'become' whatever character he needs to play through the scenes.

- If any of the scenes contain a particularly positive emotional charge for the child, suggest that you play them through again.

- At the end of the enactment, show the child how to *derole* (see 'Using drama techniques', pp.35–37), but before you do so, invite the child to say how he feels as this character, for example, 'I feel strong, clever.' 'No one can get me.' etc.

- After *deroling*, ask the child if he would like to keep anything about his character like his strength or being able to fight off dragons. Remember the child will be using metaphor in much of his play quite naturally and you do not have to, nor should you try to, interpret his thought processes.

- Equally, the child may like (or may need to be encouraged) to throw away any of the qualities he does not wish to keep, like selfishness, or controlling others.

Extensions

This sort of exercise lends itself to a commitment to paper in the form of a drawing or storyboard and can help concretize the sense of empowerment for the child.

Note of caution: It is strongly advised, if the adult is not a qualified therapist, that this exercise be used only on a single occasion, that is to say, that the child should be invited to find his 'hero within' and use the subsequent enactment as an empowerment activity only. Other internal 'heroes' can be found if further sessions are needed, but in-depth projective and role analysis work should not be attempted without training.

A BROKEN RECORD

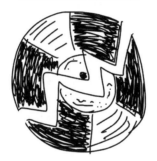

Resources

None

Application

The exercise is effective if accompanied by breathing techniques (see 'Breathing techniques', pp.145–148) and can be used on an individual or group basis.

Objectives

The aim here is to support a child who needs to stand up for himself more, for example, in bullying situations.

Exercise

- Ask the child or children if they can think of some situations where they might need to stand up for themselves, or make someone believe them, such as being wrongly blamed for something or telling someone they are being bullied or mistreated.

 – Divide the children into small groups and allow them to choose one of the situations they have described.

 – Ask them to create a small play based on the above. You can use *freeze frames* (see 'Using drama techniques', pp.35–37) or 'Beginning, Middle and End' (see 'Parental separation', pp.115–122) if the children are not able to sustain role-play.

 – Allow the children to watch and positively comment on each other's plays.

 – Discuss how the child in each play could have better stood up for himself if he had quietly repeated the same thing, for example, I *am* telling you the truth. This *is* what happened.

 – Suggest that the child concentrates on some breathing techniques prior to repeating the chosen statements and also thinks about his body language (see the activities in 'Bullying', pp.75–83).

Further activities

These may involve the use of story when the child may like to act out some favourite scenes. Suggestions for storywork are as follows:

 • *Winnie the Pooh.* As a Bear of Very Little Brain, Pooh doesn't seem to have a lot going for him and is often a favourite with children who may identify with this. Nevertheless, being popular and facing life with humour may make him a good role model and the basis for worthwhile discussion.

 • *The Ugly Duckling.* Acting out the 'ugly duckling' who is ridiculed and then hides away all winter before stepping out as a beautiful swan can be a very empowering exercise for a child, especially if performed in a group. A worthwhile discussion could then centre on each particular child's qualities and how we don't always recognize these in each other since beauty often comes from within.

Games that promote trust and eye contact which, in turn, support the development of self-esteem and confidence can be found in Appendix 2.

Other issues addressed

Anxiety, bereavement, bullying, change or transition, neglect, parental separation and sibling rivalry.

LEARNT BEHAVIOUR

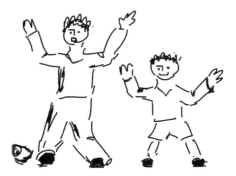

The issue

From the time a child first becomes aware of his primary carer, usually his mother, he begins to copy behaviour. The first smile, usually an event of huge delight to all, is a direct imitation of the mother's smile. From the very first, babies find human faces fascinating and attempts to contort their own faces into the same expressions can be very amusing.

In the same way, babies will try to imitate the noises around them regardless of where they come from. My eldest daughter at the tender age of one, on being asked by her grandmother about the noise 'birdies' make, came out with a loud and raucous 'Caw, Caw' since a flock of rooks had taken to settling outside her bedroom window on the telegraph wires.

Young children do not censor what they see or hear. They have no in-built faculty for deciding what is right or wrong. Consequently, when a young boy sees his father speak or act violently towards his mother, he presumes this is the way you always speak to women. This, in my experience, is becoming an issue in many schools these days where some children have difficulty in accepting discipline, especially from a female teacher.

Similarly, when a young girl sees her not-very-much older sister putting on makeup, wearing short skirts and reading about sex in teenage magazines, she presumes this is what you do when you are a girl, regardless of how young you are. The link between the early onset of puberty and sexualized behaviour has been much researched, but the fact remains that premature sexualization of children in our schools is a subject of concern to many people.

Having positive role models early in life should be a prerequisite for every child. Unfortunately, this is very often impossible for one reason or another. Once, when as a young teacher I questioned my effectiveness, I remember being told that I might well be the only positive role model these children would meet that day. It was a sobering thought. Children are like sponges and the fact that even a young girl who has been adopted, and has no biological connection to her parents, can grow up to look and sound like her adoptive mother is testimony to this fact.

The behaviours

There are many ways in which a child's behaviour may echo that of another, usually an older member of the family or family friend. Children will often grieve in the same way as their parents (see 'Bereavement', pp.66–74). At the risk of sounding sexist, it is my experience that daughters close to mothers who are in an abusive relationship will sometimes have a polarized opinion of men in general. Furthermore, sons of fathers who expect women to answer their every need immediately will expect female teachers to do the same. On the whole, however, it is, of course, impossible to generalize. Learnt behaviour is less likely to be a cross-gender issue, that is to say, sons do not normally imitate their mother's behaviour or daughters their father's.

Learnt behaviour is also very difficult to alter, especially if it is linked to a particular inherited belief system. This can be specifically true in a multi-cultural society where cultural beliefs such as suicide being an acceptable exit strategy clash with the accepted norms in the country concerned. In situations such as bereavement, a family's tradition of never talking together about issues can result in secrets and mistaken beliefs (see 'Bereavement', pp.66–74).

And occasionally a strongly held belief by a parent can produce the opposite reaction in the child. For example, a mother to whom lying is abhorrent may cross-examine her son to the extent that the son is forced to lie to defend himself.

On the whole, it is only when the child is able to form his own belief systems that learnt behaviour can be changed. Before this time the child may go through the motions of altering his behaviour to suit the circumstances at the time but will regress to indoctrinated habits if challenged. The more a child learns about the consequences of a certain behaviour as opposed to those of another, the more he will be able to make up his own mind about the way he behaves.

Activity

CONSEQUENCES

Resources

Pens
Paper
Coloured pens (optional)

Application and objectives

This activity can be used with an individual child or on a group basis. Sometimes with extreme behaviour, a useful exercise may be to do some individual work with a child first and then allow that child to 'show off' his work in front of the class, thus putting him in the position of the expert, as with the activity in 'Socially inappropriate behaviour' (pp.129–134). The overall aim of the activity is for the child to begin to make connections between action and consequence. As with any teaching aid this is best approached on a level that the child will find fun, as in the following exercise.

Exercise

– Ask the child if he would like to play a game with you. Tell him it is based on an old fashioned game called 'Consequences'.

– Say you are going to write a story each, but it is going to be muddled up.

– Give him a big piece of paper while you keep another.

– Ask him to write 'One day…' and the name of an imaginary child at the top. You do the same.

– Both fold over the top of the papers and exchange.

– Now tell the child to write down in a couple of sentences something very naughty that his character might do. You do the same.

– Fold over the papers again and exchange.

– Now write the word 'because…' and finish the sentence. (This can be left out if inappropriate to the child's age or emotional development.)

– Fold and exchange.

– Now tell the child that you are both going to write down the result of your character's naughty action.

– Exchange papers again and read out the whole story.

> *Note of caution: Care must be taken that the incongruity of the results does not detract from the seriousness of the action but rather provides a base for discussion regarding actions and possible consequences. Care should also be taken that if the subject matter becomes violent or unsociable, this is discussed appropriately.*

– Having discussed possible results of certain actions in general, one or more of the scenarios can be acted out. The child should play the part of the 'naughty child' for at least some of the time.

– Following the enactment and to leave the session on a positive note, it is worth considering with the child an alternative scenario in which his character's action achieved more pleasing results (see 'Using drama techniques: Reframing', pp.35–37).

Extensions

This exercise can be represented pictorially in addition to or instead of acting by using a storyboard. More positive actions and consequences can also be drawn in the same way.

Further activities

With older, or more emotionally developed, children it is sometimes possible to work with positive and negative role models by looking at a particular situation and discussing how one might react, first negatively and then positively, within this scenario. Both situations can then be acted out making sure that the session ends on a positive note.

Other issues addressed

Anger, bullying, compulsive lying, change or transition, parental separation, sibling rivalry and socially inappropriate behaviour.

NEGLECT

The issue

While many sources of information appear to couple the terms 'neglect' and 'abuse' together, it is my intention here to try to differentiate between the two since the sort of neglect to which I refer is that which may be defined as 'a lack of due care' which is not severe enough to require intervention by safeguarding authorities as opposed to that which is.

According to the NSPCC website, HM Government defines neglect as the persistent failure to meet a child's basic physical and/or psychological needs, likely to result in the serious impairment of the child's health or development (NSPCC 2011b). Although this definition appears clear, neglect in childhood can still be a very grey area. The borderline between what is acceptable care, and what is not, is subjective depending on culture, creed, environment and circumstances, which makes it a difficult issue to quantify, much less assess and manage. Likewise, where neglect overlaps into abuse, safeguarding authorities sometimes have a difficult job trying to collect enough evidence to act within this nebulous area. In my experience the children themselves can inhibit the process since they often have a fear that the authorities will take them away from their beloved, albeit incapable or neglectful, parent or carer.

Victoria, aged eight, was just such a child. Even though she had to sleep downstairs on the sofa with her mother in case her mother needed anything during the night, get herself up and off to school and generally do everything that her severely depressed parent could not manage, she had a vehement dislike of any outside agencies who tried to help her. Her fear of what would happen to her mother if she were not there to look after her overrode any cares she might have had for herself.

The behaviours

Children who suffer from neglect can behave in a variety of ways, ranging from being withdrawn and isolated to appearing aggressive and overly confident. Neglect often seems to breed resilience in a child as in the case of six-year-old Charlie who cheerfully looked after his two younger brothers and sisters and was sometimes late for school because he had to fetch the milk for their breakfast from the corner shop. Their mother was trying very hard to restrict her drinking and was an excellent carer when she did. At other times, on the 'bad days', Charlie filled in, happily, and as a matter of course. An outgoing, bright and bubbly child, if it weren't for his record of lateness, no one would ever guess Charlie's background.

Areas for concern

Since, as we have discussed, neglect is hard to quantify, it is obviously important to keep a written record of any areas of concern so that these can be considered as part of an overall assessment by the relevant authorities. In isolation these concerns may not constitute neglect but need to be recorded as a possible contribution to a bigger picture. Such areas may be one or more of the following:

- Failure to thrive for which no medical cause has been found.

- Developmental delay for which no medical cause has been found, especially if speech and language skills are very poor.

- Disproportionately poor academic performance, especially if coupled with poor school attendance.

- Behaviour that is abnormal for age, for example, very babyish or overly mature (especially where sexual knowledge is concerned).

- Very aggressive or very withdrawn behaviour over a substantial period of time.

- Not spending or wanting to spend time with the family or a particular family member, being nervous around or aggressive towards this person (which may indicate a fear of being hurt or a need to distance themselves).

- Excessively poor relationships with peers but constantly seeking attention from adults.

- Extreme hunger, stealing or gorging of food (in older children).

- Lack of appropriate supervision, for example, a child being left alone in the house. The NSPCC website offers guidelines on this (NSPCC 2011b).

- Physical signs of long-term neglect, for example, poor growth, protruding stomach, thinning hair and persistently cold, reddened hands and feet.

- Persistent failure by parent or carer to seek or to follow medical or nursing advice.

Activity

THE HELPER

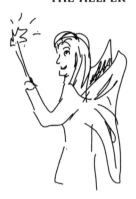

Resources

Lengths of coloured material (optional)
Dressing-up clothes (optional)
Coloured pens
Paper

Application

This exercise has been adapted from Mooli Lahad's 'Basic Ph six-part storymaking technique' (Lahad 1992) and can be used on an individual basis or with a group. There is no upper age limit since teenagers may also benefit from discovering their own inner 'helper'. A variation for use with younger children is given in 'Further activities' below.

Objectives

Very often there is little that can be done to help the child who suffers from borderline neglect, that is to say, where the situation does not warrant or for some reason is refused intervention by the relevant statutory agencies. The desirability of developing resilience in a child is controversial, but the objective of this exercise is not so much to support the 'over-resilient' child but rather to help him develop an appropriate coping mechanism which will serve him in times of hopelessness. The key to this coping mechanism lies in the nature of the helper that may be in the guise of a friend, member of the family, beloved pet, hero or heroine from a story or film or a totally fictitious character who, more often than not, embodies the crucial element of magic. For some children, for whom finding an actual helper is impossible, the acknowledgement of a 'magical' helper that represents his higher consciousness, or spiritual strength, may prove immensely supportive.

Exercise

- Explain to the child that you are going to create a fairy story together. With an older child this can be done through a short visualization when the child is invited to 'see' in his mind his hero, the mission, the obstacle, the helper and the way ahead.
- Create a short storyboard by dividing a piece of paper into six sections.
- In the first ask the child to draw his hero or heroine.
- In the second invite him to think about what it is this hero wants above anything else. (By calling this a 'fairy story' the child is encouraged to use metaphorical imagery – see 'Underpinnings of dramatherapy', pp.32–34.)
- The third will show what is stopping the hero from achieving his desires (a monster, mountain, black hole, etc.).
- The fourth (and most important) will show what or who is there to help him. (It is worth spending some time discussing this.)
- The fifth and sixth will portray the way that the hero and his helper manage to overcome the obstacles and achieve their mission and what happens in the end.
- Once the storyboard has been completed the child may then be invited to act out his story.

Extensions

The acting may precede the drawing depending on the inclination of the child.

Note of caution: Unless you are a trained therapist the above exercise should remain within the metaphor or 'story' and no attempt should be made at any interpretation or further exploitation of material. The objective here is only to support the child in finding his own mechanism for coping, not to try to bring about change.

Further activities

With a much younger child the idea of a 'helper' may be explored through the use of puppets. For example, the puppy may have a problem (which he will only tell to the child) and may need someone or thing to help him (see 'General and differentiated approaches', pp.27–28).

Other issues addressed

Anger, anxiety, bullying, change or transition, depression, lack of self-esteem/confidence, sibling rivalry and speech problems.

NIGHTMARES

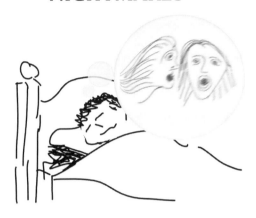

The issue

A key component of children's bad dreams is fear, which is symbolized by frightening human or non-human characters depending on the level of dreaming. This fear relates, generally speaking, to two different aspects of a child's life. One can be the difficulty he is having in reconciling the love and gentleness of the adults around him with their stricter more disciplinary traits, and/or the other, a reaction to the *actual* cruelty a child may be, or may perceive himself to be, experiencing. It has also been suggested that the wilder elements in children's dreams may symbolize those, as yet untamed, characteristics of the child himself, which are in conflict with his enforced need to follow acceptable codes of restrained behaviour.

Since children's psyches are as yet undeveloped and are constantly trying to assimilate the myriad of impressions inflicted on them every day, nightmares might be said to be a way of filtering out the tensions and anxieties invoked by these impressions and, in moderation and handled well, need not necessarily be viewed as a cause for concern but rather a natural progression in the psychic development of the child.

Most dreaming occurs in the REM (rapid eye movement) stage of sleep at the end of the night or during a period of lighter sleep. Since they are not deeply asleep, many children will wake themselves up during a nightmare, thus adding to their levels of distress and making them disinclined to want to go back to sleep.

Sometimes a child will have a nightmare following a day in which they have had a big tantrum. The 'big feelings' experienced during the tantrum are symbolized by the 'big' monsters of the dream. Being helped with the 'big feelings' in the appropriate way and at the appropriate time can calm the child and relieve the stress hormones in his brain (see 'Anger', pp.48–54).

Night terrors

A distinction needs to be made here between nightmares and *night terrors* that usually occur earlier in the night. Night terrors, described as a partial arousal from non-REM sleep, are thought to be a product of increased brain activity and can produce sweating, an increased heart beat, appearance of intense fear, crying or screaming in the child who, unlike the child suffering from a nightmare, does not remember the episode afterwards. Sometimes it is difficult to wake a child in this state, which can prove extremely distressing for the parents. They need to be reassured that more often than not night terrors disappear of their own accord and that, unless a child is sleepwalking or in danger of hurting himself, all that is needed is physical comforting and gentle reassurance. Night terrors often appear in cycles: every night for a few weeks and then nothing for a few months, and seem to occur in children whose parents or another member of the family has been a sufferer.

One intervention which has been tried with some success is to note at what time a child usually has a night terror and then to wake him about 15 minutes before that time, comfort and reassure him and send him back off to sleep.

The behaviours

Since nightmares by definition happen at night, under normal circumstances, those who care for children during the day will not necessarily be aware that a child is suffering from frequent or recurring bad dreams. The criteria for some sort of intervention lies in the words 'frequent' and/or 'recurring' since almost all children will experience nightmares at some stage of their childhood, most commonly between the ages of three and six. However, a child who is suffering from a recurring or frequent bad dream may begin to appear listless, continually tired, disinterested in work or play and may exhibit other signs of anxiety (see 'Anxiety', pp.54–58).

Recurring or frequent nightmares are usually a symptom that the child is experiencing a degree of stress, which he is unable to process properly during the hours of sleep. This may be due to an actual (or perceived) problem in the family or may even be a complete misunderstanding on the part of the child since sensitive children are prone to taking on the concerns of their elders (see 'Depression', pp.91–96) and often make mountains (or monsters) out of molehills!

Note of caution: In this situation it is obviously important to involve the parents or carers with the suggestion that they talk with their doctor about the problem. Often just talking this over with a trained professional will be enough to unblock the underlying anxiety for the child.

Activity

CHANGING THE ENDING

Resources

Pens, pencils and crayons
A4 paper
Material or dressing-up clothes (optional)

Application

Since it relates to a child's own experience it is best to use this exercise on an individual basis. However, if two children are suffering from nightmares it may be considered that, by sharing their experiences, the children will be reassured that they are not alone.

Objectives

The aim of this exercise is to replace the disturbing outcome or ending of a nightmare with a happier and more positive experience. Sometimes the 'bad ending' of a dream can replay itself in a child's mind again and again, almost seeming to take on a life of its own. By replacing this bad memory with a good one the nightmare is often laid to rest.

Note of caution: Full enactment of the nightmare should not be undertaken unless by a professional trained in this area. There is a very real danger of re-traumatization if bad experiences are re-enacted without due care. This exercise should be restricted to drawing the nightmare and only enacting the last and positive outcome.

Exercise

- Divide two pieces of paper into six or more sections.
- Invite the child to draw his nightmare as if it were a storyboard or cartoon (speech bubbles can be used if desired).
- Ask the child to look at the last frame and consider how he might like to change it so that the nightmare had a happy rather than a frightening ending (monsters overcome, etc.).
- Ask him to draw the story out again, this time with the changed ending.
- Invite the child to concentrate on the last picture and, either in a *freeze frame* (see 'Using drama techniques', pp.35–37) or by acting it out, bring this scene to life, concentrating on the feelings of empowerment for the child as he overcomes his 'demons'.

Further activities

- On the whole children do not find it helpful to have their nightmares minimized or dismissed by the words 'it was only a bad dream'. A better way to explain what has happened, in my experience, is to use the analogy of a chest of drawers where, during the day everything has been tipped out into a muddle on the floor. At night the brain is trying to sort it all out and put it back into the right drawers but sometimes it runs out of time and some things get left over. These things don't like being left out and so often turn into the monsters of the bad dreams.

- Some children like the idea of having a dream catcher, which can be hung above the head of their bed to 'catch' the bad dreams (see Appendix 3). Making a dream catcher could also be a valuable therapeutic activity for the child.

Other issues addressed

Anger, anxiety, bullying, depression, lack of self-esteem/confidence, learnt behaviour, neglect, socially inappropriate behaviour and speech problems.

PARENTAL SEPARATION

The issue

Parental separation is on the increase. The Office for National Statistics recorded that, in 2006, 23 per cent of children in Great Britain were living in lone-parent families, as opposed to 21 per cent in 1997 and 7 per cent in 1972 (Separation Statistics 2009). In the UK and Australia it is estimated that one in three marriages will end in divorce, while in the US, the figures are even higher, at approximately 45 per cent. This is only the tip of the iceberg since the figures for separating unmarried couples are much harder to come by. The divorce rate in the UK has recently fallen, but cohabitation is on the increase, and it is therefore probable that there are many more children than those recorded who are affected by their parents' separation.

In addition, one in five couples getting a divorce will already have been through one or more divorces. It is these instances of multiple changes in family organization that appear to have the most devastating effects on the children concerned.

This is not to say, however, that *every* child whose parents separate will be adversely affected. *Changing Families*, an innovative project in schools helping children from reorganized families (see Appendix 3), often comes across children for whom parental separation is a positive experience. A key issue appears to be how much support the child has at the time to understand the situation in an age-appropriate way. Help can be given to children in school to understand and come to terms with their experience while preserving the confidentiality of their parents' circumstances.

The behaviours

The presenting behaviour of children undergoing family reorganization is often very similar to that of children suffering bereavement but generally has more in common with what has been termed *complicated grief* (see 'Bereavement', pp.66–74). There is usually more confusion and misunderstanding around when families break up than when someone dies. This gives rise to feelings of guilt and blame, frustration and helplessness in addition to the sadness and anger attributed to the loss of someone or something special. Children may be inclined to take sides, blame each other, try to intervene in their parents' rows, think it's all their fault, play one parent off against another or refuse to cooperate in a reaction to their world being turned upside down and the mixed-up feelings this has invoked. Very often their feelings about what has been happening at home can isolate them at school.

In terms of the school, it is important for staff to gain an understanding of how much family circumstances can impinge on a child's ability to not only progress academically but also to develop a healthy emotional outlook on life.

Specific age-related behaviour

As in bereavement, the behaviour of children undergoing parental separation may be age-related. Younger children may regress to a time when they felt safe and their world was normal. They may become demanding, clingy or start to wet the bed again. Here again, constant reassurance and firm boundaries are necessary.

Children of school age may become insular, may be bullied or become bullies themselves. Friends may keep asking them what is wrong and a refusal to answer may result in ostracism or worse. Very often a child will not reveal what is happening at home out of loyalty to his parents, with the result that he internalizes his feelings. Sometimes this will stem from the parents themselves who regard it as 'nobody's business but theirs', little realizing that this can compound the difficulties facing their child at this time.

As with bereavement, the cycle of protection can become insidious, with parent protecting child and child protecting parent, resulting in feelings being buried and possibly causing trouble at a later date. Many children hide their real feelings not only from their parents but also from researchers, which can result in an unrealistic picture of the extent of the problem being presented.

Teenagers coming to terms with their own sexuality may suddenly be thrown into having to face that of their parents, especially if one or both parents begin a new relationship. Then the new relationship may provoke behaviour in the parent that mirrors their own in terms of flirtatiousness, sexual attraction, heightened emotions, etc. and deepen the level of confusion already being felt by the young person. In addition, teenagers may be thrown into relationships that are prematurely sexual in an effort to find someone who understands them and is there for them if their parents seem to be otherwise occupied.

Stepfamilies

In addition to the break-up of their nuclear family, children often have to cope with the sometimes sudden arrival of a new 'parent' and 'brothers and sisters'. All sorts of issues can arise, most of which have the subtext 'You don't belong here, you're not my dad/mum/brother/sister'. A child who, hitherto, had a room and toys of his own may be asked to share; adults may have different ideas of discipline or may be unfair in their treatment. Since one or all of these problems may be around for a child in school, it is hardly surprising that he fails to concentrate or sit quietly!

Desired outcomes

When working with a child from a reorganized family it may be useful to remember the following outcomes for the activities:

- To normalize the situation for the child and to help him understand that he is not alone in his feelings.
- To reassure the child that he is not babyish or silly to have these feelings.
- To support the child through the period of change or transition (see 'Change or transition', pp.83–87).
- To gently dispel any negative beliefs, for example, reason for separation, attributed blame, etc.
- To begin to enable the child to see the situation from another's viewpoint and, if appropriate, to understand motives for actions.
- To encourage the older child to take responsibility for his own actions and, if possible, to avoid conflict situations.
- To help the child form positive coping strategies and accept the new situation in his own time.

Supporting activities

- Research has shown that short-term achievable goals and tasks are most effective in dealing with children who may be suffering from a chronic low-level depression often symptomatic of children from reorganized families (see 'Depression', pp.91–96).
- Extra-curricular activities, particularly those involving physical exercise and/or group bonding, are also beneficial.

Activities

Moreover, it is advised that anyone attempting to use the following techniques restrict themselves to working within the situation as it presents itself in school rather than become involved in potentially difficult family scenarios.

Note of caution: The following activities are designed to raise awareness and support (not treat) a child going through a difficult time of parental separation. Many children require far more in-depth work than these activities offer, and need staff specially trained in this field to be able to adequately and safely address their needs as in the Changing Families project (see Appendix 3).

FAMILY PHOTO

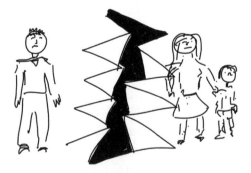

Resources
None

Application and objectives

As suggested above, a paramount objective in working with children from reorganized families is to normalize the situation and to reassure them that they are not alone. The following exercises are, therefore, best done in a group. A way of ensuring confidentiality and of allowing children to explore painful issues in a non-threatening way is to create a fictional situation. This employs a technique known as *dramatic distancing* (see 'Underpinnings of dramatherapy: Dramatic distancing', pp.32–34) whereby a child can examine his own feelings but pretend they belong to someone else (a fictional character).

Note of caution: Unless the group leader is a trained therapist this exercise should be kept within the structure of the freeze frame with sculpting and doubling techniques rather than allowing unstructured and potentially emotionally volatile improvisation or 'acting out'.

Exercise

This exercise is best done following a class or group introductory discussion about family reorganization and about how it affects so many children in schools these days.

- Tell the children you are going to create a fictional family with mum, dad and three children. (It's worthwhile exploring the meaning of 'fictional' to stress the point that this is *not* their family but a made-up one.)

- Remind the children that the family they create needs to be one that might live next door to them, that is, not a famous footballer or pop star's family.

- The technique of *hot seating* (see 'Using drama techniques', pp.35–37) is useful to flesh out the characters.

- Once the characters are in place, explore with the children why this family might be splitting up: what is causing mum and dad to argue all the time? This is a useful place to remind them that it will never be the children's fault and that it will always be adult business – usually it is because people just grow apart. Tell the children that even if these parents stop loving each other it does not mean they will stop loving their children.

- Place two chairs next to each other and invite a child to come and sit in one chair and pretend to be the dad. Ask him to sit in the way he thinks dad might sit with dad's expression on his face.

- Invite another child to come and be mum, and then each fictional child in turn.

- Ask the children doing this to consider who they think would stand close to who and why. Who might be turning away from who and why?
- When the *freeze frame* (see 'Using drama techniques', pp.35–37) is complete, invite another child to pretend to be the photographer.
- Say 'freeze' and while the family is frozen in its postures, ask another child to go around and tap each member on the shoulder. Tell the characters that when they are tapped on the shoulder they must say the first word (or sentence) that comes to mind, beginning 'I feel…'
- Use the system of *deroling* (see 'Using drama techniques', pp.35–37) to ensure that the children do not carry away with them any of their character's feelings.

Extensions

This activity can be extended into a group discussion on how this family is feeling and why. Care should be taken that it does not result in children wanting to describe their own situation at home. This can be sensitively done by always bringing the discussion back to the fictional family while acknowledging how difficult it must be for that particular child. In extreme cases it might be necessary to invite a child to come and talk to you in private after the session. (Child protection procedures should always be adhered to in these situations.)

BEGINNING, MIDDLE AND END
Resources
None

Application

This activity involves the techniques of *freeze frames*, *sculpting* and *doubling* (see 'Using drama techniques', pp.35–37).

Objectives

The objective is to elicit discussion around how arguments and difficult situations may arise in school when a family breaks up.

Exercise

- Together with a small group of children numbering between four and six, think of a situation which may be difficult for this child, for example, running away from school, becoming isolated, being bullied or bullying at school and not saying why he is upset.

- Decide who will be in the first scene, that is, where the trouble starts, and invite the children to do a *freeze frame* of the situation. Examples may be a child being bullied or interrogated about his missing father at school or a quarrel breaking out between step-siblings.
- Work out two more *freeze frames* for the middle and ending of this short story.
- Allow the three *freeze frames* to run together like a short, silent moving film.
- Make sure each child has *deroled* before returning to normal activities.
- In a group discussion afterwards, allow the children to express how they think their character was feeling and why.

Extensions

- At any point in time the group leader can shout 'freeze' and tap a character on the shoulder, asking him, as in the 'Family Photo', to complete the sentence 'I feel…'

- Alternatively the group leader may use the technique of *doubling* and, standing by a character with a hand on his shoulder, complete the sentence herself.

- *Body sculpting* can also be used to exaggerate and emphasize the emotions of the characters involved.

REFRAMING/TRYING AGAIN
Resources
Paper
Felt tip pens/crayons

Application and objectives

This exercise is interchangeable with the 'Changing the Play' exercise in 'Bullying' (pp.75–83).

This last activity should be undertaken after the preceding two when the children are used to the idea of working with *freeze frames*. Since the objective of this exercise is to turn a situation around so that it has a positive ending, improvisation can be used in the last scene to allow each character to find ways in which he can be responsible for changing the outcome. For example, understanding that a child may be upset because of a situation at home may make the teacher or other children more sympathetic.

Although this *reframing* activity may at times appear unrealistic, the aim of the exercise is to encourage each child to become aware of his own contribution to a situation and how this, even if only a word or a gesture, may be a turning or trigger point for resulting events. The emphasis is on how we can only be responsible for our own behaviour – a lesson not always learnt by adults!

Exercise

- Re-run one or more of the scenes in the previous activity.
- Discuss with the children how the 'end' scene may be more positive.
- Depending on the age and ability of the children either allow an enactment of the scene to take place while the rest of the group make suggestions by shouting 'freeze' followed by the idea (the actors will then act out the suggested idea) or discuss ideas with the group first.
- *Derole* those taking part in the enactment.
- Finish with group discussion and storyboard/cartoon drawings with speech bubbles if appropriate.

Other issues addressed

Anger, bullying, learnt behaviour and socially inappropriate behaviour.

SIBLING RIVALRY

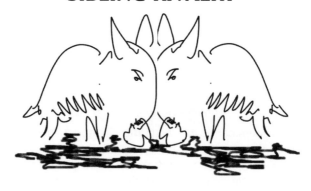

The issue

The issue of rivalry among siblings is common in families and may even start before the second child is born. In theory the problem is the province of the family and should not concern the school. In practice, however, it often does, since the emotional impact on a child can be at best disturbing and at worst devastating. As Margot Sunderland says, 'The pain of sibling rivalry with all its accompanying confusions, should never be underestimated' (Sunderland 2006, p.212). It must, therefore, be in the school's advantage for their staff to understand the major issues and age-related behaviours surrounding this common problem whether or not the school perceives it as within their remit to intervene.

On the whole most families find ways of coping with sibling rivalry, which has its roots in jealousy and competition. However, no matter how hard parents try, it is difficult for a first-born not to feel an outsider when they see the special bond between mother and baby that they remember having. This is when, as Sunderland says, they can feel '…not as lovable to my Mummy as my little sister' (2006, p.212). Sunderland also goes on to say that this feeling can influence a withdrawal of certain chemicals in the brain and the production of others resulting in aggressive behaviour and impulsivity that may start a cycle of rejection and abandonment between parent and child. Alternatively, polarization within the family may occur as one child, feeling rejected by one parent, turns to the other and forms what, in family therapy terms, is known as a 'coalition'.

Sometimes it may feel to the parents as if they are in a 'no win' situation. If they intervene in a fight between their children this may be seen as favouritism. While the 'she's younger than you' situation is often true, so too is the fact that the younger child may be the instigator, if not the bully. In circumstances where this 'favouritism' continues, the rescued child may begin to contrive the situation to their advantage. The smirk on the face of a toddler after her mother had taken her side against the viewpoint of her older children (and mine!) left me in no doubt as to just how manipulative young children can be.

Causes of sibling rivalry

The following are possible reasons why children may show signs of excessive reaction to sibling rivalry:

- Feeling threatened and not understanding the facts about the imminent arrival of a new baby, for example, mummy going to hospital, etc. (often the case with children suffering from autism or Asperger's syndrome).
- Seeking attention and being repeatedly denied it.

- Being hungry, thirsty or tired, and not having basic needs met.

- As an escape or diversion from boredom.

- Being emotionally underdeveloped: not able to differentiate between themselves and others.

- Needing an outlet for 'big feelings'.

- Attempting to assert their own identity in situations where this is denied.

- As a reaction to having a 'label' in the family, for example, the stupid one.

The behaviours

Sibling rivalry often manifests itself in constant fighting, especially in households where fighting appears to be the norm. In many cases the instigator may pick a fight as a way of getting attention from his brother or sister since he doesn't know any other way. Put-downs are also commonplace and, if not challenged, can result in some damagingly negative self-beliefs. Violence by one sibling towards another, in particular when the parent's back is turned, although not common does occur, and has been known to reach dangerous proportions in a small percentage of children.

Specific age-related behaviour

While small children may regress to babyish behaviour with the arrival of a baby in the family in the subconscious belief that this sort of behaviour attracts more attention, children of school age are more likely to react from a position of what is, and what isn't, fair. As a child's awareness of himself as others see him emerges (see 'Stages of development', pp.33–34), so too does his need to be treated equally, fairly and in the same way as others. Since the realization that life is not always fair can be devastating for some children of this age, it is worth taking time to explain how things are being dealt with as fairly as possible even though it may sometimes seem otherwise. On the whole, children will appreciate the intention even if they do not always understand the facts. An example may be when a parent has to spend more time with a sick sibling.

Teenagers who are regularly asked to shoulder more responsibility, for example, by babysitting, may become resentful of their younger brothers or sisters. This is especially so in cases of stepfamilies (see 'Parental separation', pp. 115–122).

Supporting activities

Since this is a problem that centres on the family, it is obvious that any intervention would be most effective if all the members of the family concerned were involved. The suggestion is not that school staff should intervene in family matters without appropriate training (indeed, such intervention could be ill-advised and even detrimental), but that it would be in their interest to have an understanding of the issues involved as well as some positive parenting strategies should they be in the situation of being asked for advice (see the Introduction, pp.23–37). The following points are, therefore, not intended to be used in an actively instructional way but rather to act as useful background information for the staff concerned.

- Polarization or demonization (parents or parent always blaming one child) may sometimes occur in situations where transference is present, that is, if the child reminds the parent of a relative or even of a younger version of themselves and the feelings that belong to that person are attributed to the child. 'He's just like his dad' is a common expression that speaks volumes. Parents are often less tolerant of the faults which they possessed (or possess) themselves!

- Occasionally the demonization may correlate with the parent's expectations of that child which, in turn, may have its roots in the parent's own unfulfilled ambitions.

- Sibling rivalry may be more intense when siblings are of the same gender and are close in age.

- Basic household ground rules that can be agreed by the family, written up and displayed are a useful resource in times of dispute.

- Quick intervention or 'rescuing' on the part of the parent can, as we have seen, result in favouritism and manipulation issues. Separating the fighting siblings and allowing time for feelings to subside before calmly discussing the problem is a much better strategy.

- Spending too much time attributing blame is often counter-productive. 'It takes two to tangle' is true more often than not.

- More constructive might be to take the opportunity to teach the life skills of negotiation, compromise and conflict resolution.
- Quiet, focused, 'special' time (ideally involving play) as often as possible for each child alone with the parent can be very beneficial.

Areas for concern

Much of the above may not be apparent in school life but may become a problem if, for example, siblings meet in the playground or in after-school clubs. Individual mood and temperament will obviously play a major part in each child's reaction but schools should become concerned if the rivalry appears to be escalating into the realms of physical, emotional or sexual abuse (see 'Abuse', pp.42–48 and 'Depression', pp.91–96) or if the child concerned becomes unnaturally withdrawn or aggressive.

Activities

BABES IN THE WOOD

Resources
Lengths of coloured material
Pebbles or small stones

Application
This activity is best used when there is known animosity or rivalry between two siblings. (It has also been used effectively for children who are not siblings.)

Objective
The objectives are, through the metaphor, to encourage the children to explore what they have in common rather than their differences and how they can support each other against a third party.

Exercise
- Read, tell or remind the children of the story *Babes in the Wood*.
- Either allow the children to enact the whole story with the group leader playing the parts of the father, wicked stepmother and witch, or pick certain scenes to show a beginning, middle and end.
- After the enactment, discuss and enact other ways in which the children, as the 'babes', could outwit the evil witch or stepmother.

Extensions

Depending on the age and cognitive ability of the children, this exercise could be extended into looking at different ways in which children can support each other against other perceived hostile encounters, for example, bullies, neighbourhood gangs, etc.

THE DESERT ISLAND

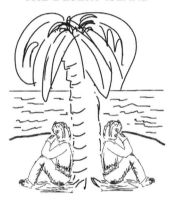

Resources

Lengths of coloured material
Dressing-up clothes (optional)
Clay
Length of wallpaper
Felt tip pens/crayons

Application

This exercise can be used with two or more children who are not getting on regardless of whether or not they are siblings. Depending on the level of imagination and engagement, this exercise could extend over a series of sessions. A large room is necessary to make this exercise successful.

Objective

The objective is for the children to learn the need for skills of negotiation and compromise in a creative and playful way.

Exercise

– Ask the children to imagine they have been shipwrecked onto a desert island.

- Here you might like to create the island using material, chairs, cushions, etc. and explore its main topographical features: rivers, mountains or even volcanoes and dangerous swamps or jungles.
- Explain that there is fresh water on the island but it is half a day's walk away and they have nothing to carry it in as yet.
- Tell the children that they must decide certain things: if they need a leader, and if so, who will it be; where they will live; what they will do for food.
- Invite them to make up a name for their group.
- Tell them that, in order to survive, they have to make up certain rules for their group.
- Depending on the group allow the children as much free rein as possible to manage their own survival.
- From time to time, add instructions or comments such as, 'It is now growing dark, you must get together everything you need to survive the night.' 'There is a sail appearing on the horizon.' 'A very large crocodile has just emerged from the swamp.' 'There are signs that the volcano is beginning to erupt.' etc.
- After issues of leadership, compromise, negotiation, teamwork, reaction to stress, etc. have been explored through the metaphor, a 'rescue' can be engineered.
- *Derole* the children so that they do not carry over the fantasy into the classroom (see 'Using drama techniques', pp.35–37).

Extensions

- This exercise may be preceded or followed up with a craft activity such as making the island out of clay.
- Depending on the cognitive and emotional age of the group, the exercise may be brought into reality and the actual issue of the children's dissension discussed. Strategies for conflict resolution may then evolve.

Further activities

- Group games that encourage or necessitate teamwork will be useful here and may be a good way to start or finish a session (see Appendix 1).

- Alternative scenarios may be invented which may be more age-appropriate such as 'Escape from a Prison of War Camp' for teenagers. These scenarios may involve more detailed planning.

Note of caution: Bringing these exercises out of the metaphor and into reality admits the potential of disclosure. An awareness of the school's child protection procedure is obviously a prerequisite to this work.

Other issues addressed

Anxiety, bullying, lack of self-esteem/confidence, learnt behaviour, neglect and socially inappropriate behaviour.

SOCIALLY INAPPROPRIATE BEHAVIOUR

The issue

There are many reasons why a child may display socially inappropriate behaviour. Perhaps the most common of these is an autistic disorder, which often manifests itself as a lack of social awareness. Children suffering from autism or Asperger's syndrome often appear as emotionally withdrawn or unavailable. They seem unable to connect on a deeply human level and often do not respond in socially acceptable ways. Much has been written on the subject of autism and much research has been done into looking at effective interventions. There are also conflicting professional views as to the diagnosis of autism which are not appropriate for discussion here. Suffice it to say that autism is often difficult to diagnose and should be left to an educational or clinical psychologist.

Learnt behaviour, or behaviour that is copied from another (usually a member of the family), can also be the cause of a child behaving in a socially unacceptable manner. This most often manifests itself in swearing, bullying, violent or aggressive behaviour but may also be the reason behind prematurely sexual behaviour (see 'Learnt behaviour', pp.103–106) or issues in grieving (see 'Bereavement', pp.66–74). It may also be the case that the child's upbringing, although not reprehensible in itself, has not adequately equipped the child for social interaction in the outside world.

The fact remains, however, that whatever the diagnosis, a child who is exhibiting socially inappropriate behaviour needs support, and the following suggestions and activities are offered as applicable to any child who is finding it difficult to fit into the world around him, for whatever reason.

The behaviours

Many of the ways in which we can recognize a child who has trouble in behaving in a socially appropriate manner involve friendship issues. Children are often unforgiving when it comes to measuring how well one of their peers fits into the crowd. On the whole they are much more likely to take a physical disability in their stride than a child who appears strange to them. A little boy I knew who was the only son of very loving and demonstrative parents, and who had little social interaction with children he knew outside school, was shunned by his classmates who described him as 'weird'. He did not realize that not everyone likes to receive 'butterfly kisses' (brushing eyelashes against the cheek), especially in front of a class.

Socially inappropriate behaviour, therefore, often manifests itself in one or more of the following ways:

- Inappropriate use of body language and space. Some children do not have an awareness of what is socially acceptable in terms of close contact or gestures. This may be due to a different cultural upbringing, as what is acceptable in one society is not necessarily so in another, and this should always be taken into account before chastising a child for what seems abnormal behaviour.

- Lack of empathy. Some children who have had an unresponsive upbringing (see 'Lack of self-esteem/confidence', pp.96–102) simply do not have an understanding of what another child may be feeling. This may lead to difficulties in social interactions, especially if the child appears to be uncaring or show no remorse over something he has done. It is always worthwhile considering in these cases whether the child is actually *capable* of understanding how another feels before chastising him for not doing so.

- Inability to understand the social cues of other children. Some children's timing appears to be an issue in their interactions with others. They may miss cues, which means they jump in too quickly with an inappropriate remark, or appear to be sullen by not responding when in reality they are not sure how to react.

Activities

THE ALIEN PUPPET

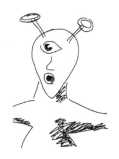

Resources
Two different puppets

Application
This exercise is best done on a one-to-one basis so that the child's ideas can be followed up and the delicate process of projection (see 'Underpinnings of dramatherapy: Stages of development', pp.32–34) played through. Any two puppets can be used, providing they are quite different in character, especially if one is slightly stranger looking than the other.

Objective
The purpose of this exercise is for the child to teach himself the way to behave since it is necessary for him to make the connection in his brain between what others are telling him to do and what he, himself, intrinsically knows is right. Children with learning difficulties in particular seem to have a problem with this.

Exercise
– Tell the child that one of the puppets (perhaps the strange looking one) has come from another planet. Think up a name for the puppet. Say that sometimes [name] finds it difficult to understand how people on Planet Earth behave. (You may like to play out the puppet's arrival on Earth.)

- Explore together what this puppet does. Allow the child to lead in this by having the alien puppet. Keep your critical responses as the other puppet to a minimum but suggest every now and again that this is not what people do on Planet Earth. Remember the child's ideas.

- Suggest you swap puppets. With the alien puppet repeat the child's actions and ideas but exaggerate these so that the behaviour appears even stranger.

- When the child tells you, through the other puppet, how to behave, use your own judgement as to whether to ignore his advice at first (encouraging the child to become angry or irritable or more forceful, reactions which he would have provoked in real life). Always finish, however, by taking the advice.

- If appropriate you may wish to invite the child to run through one last scenario in which the alien puppet has learnt how to behave on Planet Earth. How do people around him react to him now? How does he feel about this?

This activity may need to be performed over a number of sessions until the message goes home!

ME IN MY BUBBLE

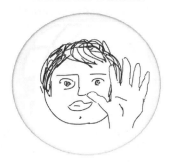

Resources
None

Application and objectives
This activity addresses the issue of awareness of one's own space in relation to others and should be performed in a group of not less than six children. It can be used with a whole class to encourage spatial awareness, empathy and group appreciation and has various stages, the final one of which is a game which most children love.

Exercise

Stage 1: Awareness of space

- Ask the children to stand in a space in the room where they can spread their arms wide and imagine themselves inside a bubble.
- Ask them to move slowly at first around the room, making sure that their bubble does not collide with anyone else's. (With older children you may wish to allow them to go only forwards, sideways, backwards, etc.)

Stage 2: Awareness of others

- At any given point, shout 'stop' and ask them to close their eyes.
- Ask them, without opening their eyes, to point to where they think [a member of the group] is standing.
- When everyone has pointed, ask them to open their eyes to see how right they were.
- With a small group make sure everyone has a turn at being pointed at.

Stage 3: Group awareness

- Ask the children to begin moving around in their bubbles like before.
- Tell them that this time you are not going to shout 'stop' but you are simply going to stop moving. When you stop they have to. They must be aware of where you are at all times but not simply follow you. The objective is to see how quickly the members of the group can sense you stopping and stop moving themselves.
- Allow everyone in a small group to have a go at being the leader and stopping the group.

Stage 4: Group awareness game

- Tell the children that you are going to turn this exercise into a game.
- Invite one child to go outside the door to be the 'detective'.
- While the detective is outside, pick another child to lead and stop the group.
- The objective of the game is for the detective to guess who is stopping the group. Obviously the more aware the group are of each other the more quickly they will stop and the more difficult it will be for the detective to come up with the right person.

Further activities

Further games for groups, which encourage social awareness, can be found in Appendix 1.

Other issues addressed
Bullying, lack of self-esteem/confidence and learnt behaviour.

SPEECH PROBLEMS
The issue

Note of caution: This section is only intended to be applicable for children whose problems with speech are either so slight as to not require referral or who are awaiting referral to a qualified speech and language therapist. Under no circumstances should the activities be deemed to replace professional advice.

Most sources of research agree that speech and language problems affect about 5 per cent of children of school age. Although this does not seem to be a huge proportion, being unable to communicate in an appropriate way may have long-term affects on a child, not only in terms of his academic progress but also his social-emotional development. Loss of hearing is less likely these days to go undetected and therefore to continue to be a cause although it may still be a problem in some areas. Occasionally I still come across the young child who has been labelled as 'difficult', 'in his own world' or who 'refuses to take any notice' when the truth is he doesn't actually *hear* what anyone else is saying.

There are many reasons why a child may have difficulty in making himself understood: these may be physiological, genetic, developmental (possibly linked to other disabilities causing delays), neurological (different processing in the brain) or emotional. It is also possible that an increase in speech problems among children may be linked to too much time being spent in front of the TV or computer screen: the incessant noise produced being detrimental to the natural development of speech and language skills. Whatever the reason, having a child who cannot easily communicate in a class of 30 or so other children can be a problem for school staff and, while awareness of the need for more speech and language therapists is growing, there remains, at least in my part of the world, a substantial shortfall in this area.

The behaviours

Under normal circumstances most children have learnt to speak in a language, the major part of which can be understood by the age of five. This development can be spasmodic: not all children learn to speak at the same rate and not all children develop their sentence construction (language skills) and articulation of sounds (speech skills) in a uniform manner. For example a five-year-old child may be talking in long sentences but may not be understood because the sounds he is making are unclear.

Between the ages of two and five it is normal for a child to repeat words and phrases, to stammer and to use hesitation, saying 'um' or 'er' while he is trying to sort out what he wants to say. However, if by the age of four a child is still using repetition and is showing no signs of spontaneous speech, if he has problems communicating through language what he wants, if his speech is causing him to be teased or bullied, or if he still cannot be mostly understood by strangers, then there should be some cause for concern and the appropriate professionals should be contacted for an assessment.

Specific difficulties may include an inability to put words in the right order in a sentence or enunciating certain words or sounds. Stammering (known also as stuttering) may also affect some children but it is worth remembering that while many will go through a period of stammering (between the ages of two and five children often repeat words and phrases) three-quarters of them will recover, and only about 1 per cent will have a long-term problem. Even then, as many famous people such as Julia Roberts and Bruce Willis (not to mention Colin Firth in the film 'The King's Speech'!) can testify, stammering can be overcome with adequate support and motivation.

Supporting activities

The following are some general tips for dealing with a child with speech and language problems:

- Maintain eye contact and if possible come down to his level.

- Slow down your own speech and find the appropriate level for his age.

- Be patient and never correct his grammar.

- Use a running commentary if you are doing something while he is watching to allow him to hear appropriate language in a relaxed way.

- Use songs and rhymes in a fun way with him (speech impediments often improve or are non-existent when singing or reciting rhyme).

Activities

DIVING FOR LANDS

Resources

Length of coloured material
Cushions
Dressing-up clothes (optional)

Application

Most children up to about the age of ten (and sometimes older) will enjoy this activity which can be used on an individual basis but is much more fun with three or four. The room needs to be of a reasonable size and if possible, have curtains or blinds that can be shut, thus making the whole adventure more exciting.

Objective

The objective of this exercise is to provide a scenario which is both liberating and fun so that, in the 'heat of the moment', the child may overcome any hesitancies or fears about expressing himself correctly.

Exercise

- Explain to the child that you are going to pretend to go on an adventure to another 'land' and that he can choose where to go. (This will depend on the fabric/materials available and the imagination of others taking part.)

- A child, 'the traveller', stands on a cushion and says: 'I want to go to [a country of his choice]'. He then makes a dive into a pile of cushions or material.

- While the traveller buries his head and counts (say up to fifty), the rest of the group draws the curtains and transforms the room into the chosen land.

- When the land is ready the child is invited to open his eyes and is escorted over some stepping-stone cushions into the adventure.

- Everyone in the new land speaks in a foreign language and the traveller is encouraged to do so too.
- When the adventure is finished, the child is escorted back over the stepping-stones and covers his eyes again while the room is changed back into its original state.

Extensions

The adventure can then be discussed with all the children. It is part of the 'magic' for the traveller to recount his adventure and for the rest of the group to feign surprise. This is the 'willing suspension of disbelief', and it is important to the healthy psychological and emotional development of the child (see 'Preface: Why drama?', pp. 17–22).

TALKING IN NUMBERS

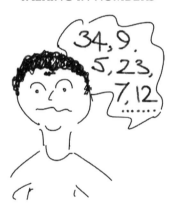

Resources
None

Application

This exercise is best used with at least two or three children and with those over the age of about seven who are capable of understanding body language.

Objective

As in the preceding exercise, the objective here is to allow the fun of the game to overcome the child's nervousness at expressing himself. By taking away the necessity to make himself understood in recognizable language and using numbers (or a foreign language) instead, the child is empowered to communicate more freely.

Exercise

- Explain to the children that you are going to play a guessing game. Two of you are going to have a conversation but not in words: you will be using numbers instead.

- With one child think of an easy situation, for example, a mother scolding her child for being late, a child wanting his mum or dad to buy him something, a teacher first being exasperated and then pleased with a child's work, a child being bullied and then standing up for himself.

- Using only numbers and plenty of gestures/body language, mime the short scene. (You may have to take the leading part at first.) For example, instead of saying 'I want some sweeties' say '5, 8, 2' or '24, 35, 64'. It doesn't matter what numbers you use, it is the tone of voice that matters, not the words.

- The other child/rest of the group have to guess what they think is happening.

Extension

Instead of using numbers, the words may be sung to a familiar tune.

Further activities

One-word stories can be used to allow the child to slow down his speech and emphasize one word at a time. Take it in turns with the child to say a word and see what story emerges. A variation on this is to mime the story as it emerges. This could be extended into a class activity with children in pairs rehearsing their story to show to the others. (This variation should not be used if it induces a stress reaction in the child with the speech impediment.)

Other issues addressed

Anxiety and lack of self-esteem/confidence.

TRAUMA AND SHOCK

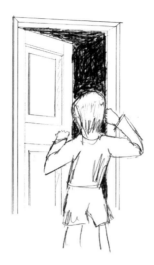

The issue

There are many reasons why a child of school age may be experiencing a state of shock, stress or, at the sharp end of the scale, trauma, most commonly PTSD. One of the increasingly widespread causes is the uncontrolled and unmeasured viewing or witnessing of violence. This commonly involves either access to inappropriate material in the form of excessively violent films, DVDs, computer games, etc. or real-life violence and abuse within the home or community. Also in a recent study of 268 serious case reviews, the NSPCC found that domestic abuse was a risk factor in 34 per cent. Furthermore it was discovered that 12 per cent of under 11's, 18 of 11–17's and 24 per cent of 18–24 year olds had been exposed to domestic abuse between adults in their homes during childhood (www.nspcc.org.uk/inform/research/statistics/domesticabusewda87794htlm, accessed on 9 March 2012).

The behaviours

It is estimated that about two-thirds of every assault within the home is witnessed by a child. The effect on the child is dependant on various factors, for example, the nature of the violence witnessed, the length or frequency of the exposure, the developmental stage of the child, etc. Depending on the latter and the nature of the child, he may mirror the witnessed behaviour, assuming that an angry and aggressive style of conduct is not only acceptable but the norm. His potential arousal to aggressive situations is heightened while the likelihood of his being able to use restraint is diminished. The child can become desensitized to violence, resulting in a decreased ability to empathize with the pain or distress of others.

The permanent threat of sudden violence can lead a child to become hypervigilant. At the slightest provocation, stress hormones will flood the brain and body, resulting in hyperactivity, anxiety and impulsive behaviour. His ability to learn and to develop emotional intelligence will also be affected, as will his propensity to play and explore.

There are various coping strategies which children employ to lessen the intensity of trauma, stress or shock. These include hypervigilance (always being in a state of alert in case something happens), projection (pretending that what is happening is happening to someone else), splitting (inventing a part of themselves that is able to cope with the trauma and giving it a form) or straightforward denial.

During a traumatic incident a child will become helpless. Normally they are unable to fully grasp what is going on and feel totally out of control. If they are unable to do anything about what is going on they will automatically go into a fight/flight/freeze response. Dr. Peter Levine, an international authority on healing trauma, tells us that after trauma bodies are meant to return to normal after this adrenaline rush. When this restorative process is thwarted, the trauma remains embedded in the mind or body and the person becomes traumatized. In nature, he tells us, an impala will resort to a 'freezing' response when threatened by a cheetah. Once (if he is lucky and the cheetah decides to look elsewhere for its prey) the danger is past, the impala will come out of its 'frozen' state, shake off the residual energy and carry on as if nothing had happened (Levine 1997). Unfortunately for humans, and especially for children, this is not so easy. Children may experience many events that are not necessarily life threatening, but whether they are or not, the effect on their coping mechanisms is the same: overwhelming. This residual energy does not (as Levine tells us) simply vanish. Remaining in the body it can give rise to a variety of complaints such as depression, pervading anxiety and all sorts of other psychosomatic (manifested in the body) symptoms. The problem is that the parts of the brain that are activated by trauma are the lower (instinctual) brain and the limbic (emotional) brain, which are the parts we share with animals. The higher or human part of the brain, which might bring a calmer, more rational reaction, is not involved.

Areas for concern

It is usually the presence of one or more of the following behaviours *occurring without demonstrative cause* that might uphold the consideration that exposure to witnessed violence may be associated:

- Repetitive play.
- Continual state of hypervigilance or high activity level, easily distracted.
- Numbing and inability to comfort self.
- Bed wetting and/or nightmares.
- Intense anxiety disorders, panic attacks or phobias.
- Dissociation.
- Flashbacks (repetitive experiencing of a particularly disturbing scene), usually visual.
- Play involving high levels of aggression or coercion of others.

Note of caution: Children suffering from trauma or shock and who are displaying one or more of the behaviours above will require the trained help and support of a suitably qualified and experienced therapist. There are no activities that I would consider safe to suggest beyond those aimed at raising levels of self-esteem and confidence (see 'Lack of self-esteem/confidence', pp.96–102) and 'Trust activities' (see 'Attachment', pp.58–65). Even the activity that is aimed at differentiating between fact and fantasy (see 'Compulsive lying: Fibs and Fact', pp.87–91) should not be used where there is known to be actual domestic violence.

CONCLUSION

WHAT TO DO AT THE END OF A SESSION
Closure activities

It is worthwhile giving some thought as to how you are going to end a session which may have dealt, even if only insignificantly, with emotional issues. The safe, nurturing environment that may have been fostered during this time may well be vastly different from the noisy canteen or challenging classroom. A few minutes spent in a calming or reassuring activity may be time well spent since it will help this transition and may avoid a child expressing his discomfort through anger 'blips' or tantrums.

At the end of any session it is important that the individual child or children return to their normal activities in as calm and controlled a manner as possible. To do this it may be necessary to repeat a familiar routine or perform a ritualistic action or activity, which, to the child, signals the end of the session. Sometimes this may be as simple as putting away the material used together. However you end the session it is not a good idea to do so abruptly and without warning. It is enough to say, 'We shall have to think of an ending to this story/game, etc. now because we have to stop in five/ten minutes.'

Occasionally, with an especially vulnerable child it may be necessary to accompany him into the classroom and remain with him for a short while, helping him re-engage with his academic work.

Closure activities may take the form of breathing exercises or visualizations (see 'Calming activities', pp.145–148) or may be group acknowledgement or massage exercises. The following are examples of activities suitable for use with a group of children.

Group massage

> Note of caution: To comply with current legislation it is advised that all physical contact be between the children themselves, with adults only directing the activities without becoming involved.

THE MOTORWAY

- Ask the children to stand in a circle and then all turn to their right so that they can place their hands on the shoulders of the child in front.
- Tell them you are all going to build a motorway.
- Begin by clearing away the rubble by smoothing hands down over the backs from neck to waist, taking in the arms.
- Next slap on the tarmac in gentle patting motions all over the shoulders and upper back.
- Smooth down the tarmac by using firm strokes up the back and over the shoulders.
- Run two fingers down either side of the backbone to draw the centre lines in the road.
- Run the fingers gently and very lightly from the top of the head down and over the whole upper part of the body. (This is the rain shower or sprinklers to cool the tarmac!)

Group acknowledgement activities

A group will have a life of its own and one that has built up a degree of mutual trust will sometimes go through a period of mourning at the end of the sessions. With older children what they have gained from being part of a group can be expressed verbally, for example, in rounds of 'What I liked best/least was…' and 'What I'm taking away/leaving behind is…', but with younger children this needs to be acknowledged more symbolically.

The following are ideas for ending sessions.

TANGLES

- With a group of not more than about 12 children ask them to hold hands across the circle. They should hold the hands of two different people.
- Once everyone has found a hand to hold, say that they are now going to try to untangle themselves. They may need to step over or under arms so need to be careful.

- Once the group is standing back in a circle holding hands, ask them to pass a squeeze around.

SAY MY NAME LIKE…

- One child stands in the middle of the circle and says, 'Say my name like [a waterfall, a loud drum, fireworks, chocolate, etc.].'
- This involves a degree of imagination on the part of the group who continue to say the name in the required fashion for a few minutes, during which time the child in the middle can close his eyes.
- With younger children it may be necessary to restrict the choice to 'loudly, softly, quickly, slowly' or a combination of any of these.

CLOSE EYES AND POINT

- This exercise is a variation on Stages 1 and 2 of 'Me in my Bubble' (see 'Socially inappropriate behaviour', pp.129–134). Ask the children to begin to move slowly around the room in any direction they wish, being careful not to knock into each other.
- At a given point say 'Stop. Close your eyes and point to where you think…is.'
- When the children open their eyes again they can point in the correct direction chanting the name of the child in question three or four times. (Much cheating usually goes on here but the objective is for each child to be acknowledged rather than for the pointing to be accurate.)

Calming activities

Breathing techniques

Note of caution: Always insisting that the children breathe in through their noses and not their mouths diminishes the potentiality for them to hyperventilate. No deep breathing technique should be continued over a long period of time. Building up a regular practice in short intervals is most advisable.

THE WOODCHOPPER

Both this exercise and 'The Saucepan' exercise (see Anger, pp.48–54) focus on expelling the pent-up energy of tension, anger or anxiety and are best used, if necessary, before any other more calming technique.

- Tell the children you are all going to safely chop up a big log.
- Ask them to imagine this log in front of them on the ground and that they are holding a large axe in both hands.
- Ask them to raise it above their heads as they take a big breath in through their nose.
- As they expel the breath with a loud noise through their mouth they bring down the axe to chop up the log.
- Repeat up to ten times.

Note of caution: If you feel that using an axe is inappropriate for some children who may abuse the idea, the imagery may need to be change to something less violent, for example, blowing up a balloon, etc.

BELLY BREATHING

This technique is a good introduction to explain to children how, generally speaking, we only use the top parts of our lungs and that to be really healthy we need to breathe deeply.

- Make sure every child is sitting comfortably in an upright chair with both feet on the floor and hands in their laps.
- It is helpful to ask children either to close their eyes or focus on some object placed in the middle of the circle. (Be aware that children who have suffered some sort of abuse often find it too scary to close their eyes or be blindfolded.)
- Ask the children to put their hands on their stomach with the tips of the fingers touching.
- Ask them to take a very deep breath in through their nose and feel the air travelling down through their lungs and making their stomach rise.
- As their stomach rises ask them to notice how their fingers come apart.
- Now tell them to let their stomach sink, the fingers come back together again and ask them to notice the breath travelling back up through the lungs and out through their nose.

This technique, derived from the complete breath of yoga, takes some practice, and very young children often find it impossible, in which case 'Candle Breathing' (see below) may be more appropriate.

ONE, TWO, THREE, FOUR

As a follow-on to 'Belly Breathing' the technique below may be used:

- Tell the children they are going to breathe in and out through their nose.
- Say that you are going to count in and out slowly: to the count of four.
- Count 'In, two, three, four' and 'Out, two, three, four' at a pace you feel is right for the children. It is better to start at a reasonable pace and then slow it down as the children (and their lungs) become used to the practice.

Variation: With older children, especially those who are preparing for exams and who may benefit from a calming and de-stressing activity, the counts may be extended to five, six or even eight. Begin by slowly lengthening the out breath first. Another extension is to adopt the yoga practice of acknowledging the spaces in between the breaths as a prelude to achieving a level of stillness, which is a prerequisite to the practice of meditation. A ratio often used in yoga practices is as follows:

- Breathe in, two, three, four…
- Hold breath, two three, four…
- Breathe out, two, three, four…
- Hold breath, two, three, four…

Note of caution: Do not attempt to extend the above counts until the young person can manage these properly.

GORILLA BREATHING

Another technique derived from yoga focuses on bringing oxygen to both hemispheres of the brain and encouraging them to work together. Called alternate nostril breathing in yoga, it has been named gorilla breathing to help the child visualize the swinging of the arms up to block each nostril in turn.

- Ask the children to sit comfortably and imagine that they have the long arms of a gorilla.
- Explain that they are going to breathe in and out of each side of their nose in turn to help their brain get enough oxygen on both sides.
- Ask them to swing their right arm up and with the first finger of the right hand, block the right nostril.
- Breathe in through the left nostril, keeping the right one blocked.

- Swing up the left arm and block the left nostril with the first finger.
- Swing down the right arm and breathe out through the right nostril, keeping the left one blocked.
- Breathe in through the right nostril, keeping the left one blocked.
- Swing up the right arm, block the right nostril and breathe out of the left nostril, keeping the right one blocked.
- Breathe in through the left nostril, keeping the right one blocked, etc.

Note: Remembering that the in breath follows the out breath *in the same nostril* may make this easier. Plenty of tissues are needed for this exercise!

CANDLE BREATHING (FOR YOUNGER CHILDREN)

For very little children breathing in and out of their nose is often difficult. It is also much easier for them to have something simple and familiar to visualize in order to help them concentrate.

- Tell the children to put up a first finger in front of their face and imagine it is the flame of a candle.
- Ask them to take a big breath in through their nose if possible.
- Ask them to breathe gently out through their mouth, making the candle flame flicker but not go out.
- Gently extend the out breath by counting to four, then five, etc.

Visualizations

A guided visualization either with or without suitable music is a way of ending a session, which most children enjoy. With a few provisos, visualizations, which are empowering, positive, uplifting and nurturing, can be written by staff or even the children themselves. (Older children often like to do this for younger ones.) Care should obviously be taken not to refer to anything that might be frightening or threatening, for example, dark woods, high places, rough seas or deep pools. Words that conjure up the idea of light, happiness and safety should be emphasized. On the whole it is best not to include people in visualizations unless it is prefaced by something like, 'someone you know who loves you'.

Examples of visualizations that work best are those that the children conjure up mostly for themselves, for example, 'the circle of friends' or 'the safe place'. In both visualizations the child imagines beloved, safe, familiar objects or people around them which or who will always be there whenever he needs them.

More suggestions for using visualizations are given in Appendix 3.

Appendix 1
GROUP BONDING GAMES

The following are some examples of games that can be used to help children function well as a group. For any sort of group that has as its objective emotional support, it is important that a level of trust and cooperation between group members is achieved before any sort of mutually supportive work can be done. Some ideas for trust exercises are given in 'Attachment' (pp.58–65) but the following exercises focus more on an optimum level of cooperation and performance.

THE ADVERB GAME
This game is for children from about age nine upwards.
- Divide the children into groups of four or five.
- Each group will take it in turns to think of an adverb. This may need the explanation of 'how you do something', for example, carefully, slowly, happily, etc.
- Each group will take a turn of being 'on stage'.
- The audience will shout action words at the group, for example, 'running', 'swimming', 'washing a car', 'climbing a ladder', etc.
- The group on stage will perform the action in the manner of the adverb they have chosen, for example, 'happily climbing a ladder'.
- The audience has to guess the adverb.

GROUP MIME
- Divide the children into groups of three, four or five.
- Give each group a mime to perform. Suggestions might be 'herding a flock of sheep down a busy street on market day', 'moving a grand piano up a flight of stairs' or 'washing an elephant'.

- Each group has to work together to perform their mime for the audience to guess.

PARTS OF THE BODY

- Explain to the children that each part of the body counts for a different number. For example, feet are both 1, hands are both 5 and bottoms are 2.
- Divide the children into small groups.
- Say a number and see if the group can work it out so that they have body parts representing that number touching the floor.
- Occasionally this may mean members supporting each other or lifting each other off the floor.

Variations: Vary the numbers in the group or the body parts.

Appendix 2
INDEX OF ISSUES AND SUPPORTING ACTIVITIES

Abuse: The Shield; Trust exercises; In the Mirror; Calming activities.

Anger: Mr. Angry Man; The Volcano; The Saucepan; Trust exercises; You May Think...; The Dragon Story; Opposite Corners; Consequences; Changing the Ending; Calming activities; Beginning, Middle and End; Reframing/Trying Again.

Anxiety: Ben's Bag of Worries; Mr. Angry Man; The Helper; The Volcano; The Saucepan; The Shield; In the Mirror; 'I Need You to Listen'; Trust exercises; The Divided Room; Opposite Corners; My Hero; Changing the Ending; Babes in the Wood; Talking in Numbers; Diving for Lands; Calming activities.

Attachment: Back to Back; Push Hands; Group Fall; Jailers; 1, 2, 3; Trust exercises; The Shield; My Hero.

Bereavement: You May Think...; The Dragon Story; Ben's Bag of Worries; Mr. Angry Man; Trust exercises; The Saucepan; The Volcano; The Shield; The Two Islands; Opposite Corners; My Hero; Calming activities.

Bullying: The Status Game/I'm OK; In the Mirror; 'I Need You to Listen'; Changing the Play; Ben's Bag of Worries; Mr. Angry Man; The Volcano; The Saucepan; The Shield; Trust exercises; Opposite Corners; A Broken Record; My Hero; Consequences; The Helper; Changing the Ending; Beginning, Middle and End; Reframing/Trying Again; The Desert Island; Babes in the Wood; Me in my Bubble; Calming activities.

Change or transition: The Two Islands; Ben's Bag of Worries; Mr. Angry Man; You May Think...; The Dragon Story; Trust exercises; In the Mirror;

The Status Game; 'I Need You to Listen'; Changing the Play; Opposite Corners; My Hero; Consequences; The Helper; Calming activities.

Compulsive lying: The Divided Room/Fibs and Fact; Trust exercises; Consequences; Calming activities.

Depression: Opposite Corners; The Shield; Mr. Angry Man; In the Mirror; Trust exercises; The Helper; Changing the Ending; Calming activities.

Lack of self-esteem/confidence: My Hero; A Broken Record; The Status Game; In the Mirror; 'I Need You to Listen'; Changing the Play; Ben's Bag of Worries; The Shield; Trust exercises; The Two Islands; The Divided Room; Opposite Corners; The Helper; Changing the Ending; Babes in the Wood; Me in my Bubble; Diving for Lands; Talking in Numbers; Calming activities.

Learnt behaviour: Consequences; Trust exercises; In the Mirror; 'I Need You to Listen'; Changing the Play; Changing the Ending; Beginning, Middle and End; The Desert Island; Reframing/Trying Again; The Alien Puppet; Calming activities.

Neglect: The Helper; Ben's Bag of Worries; The Shield; Trust exercises; My Hero; A Broken Record; Changing the Ending; Babes in the Wood; The Desert Island; Calming activities.

Nightmares: Changing the Ending; Ben's Bag of Worries; Mr. Angry Man; The Saucepan; Trust exercises; The Divided Room; Calming activities.

Parental separation: Family Photo; Beginning, Middle and End; Reframing/Trying Again; Ben's Bag of Worries; Mr. Angry Man; The Volcano; The Saucepan; Trust exercises; The Two Islands; Opposite Corners; A Broken Record; My Hero; Consequences; Calming activities.

Sibling rivalry: Babes in the Wood; The Desert Island; Ben's Bag of Worries; Mr. Angry Man; Trust exercises; Consequences; Calming activities.

Socially inappropriate behaviour: The Alien Puppet; Me in my Bubble; In the Mirror; The Status Game; 'I Need You to Listen'; Trust exercises; My Hero; A Broken Record; Calming activities; Consequences; The Helper; Changing the Ending; Beginning, Middle and End; Reframing/Trying Again; The Desert Island.

Speech problems: Diving for Lands; Talking in Numbers; Ben's Bag of Worries; The Helper; Changing the Ending; Calming activities.

Trauma and shock: Calming activities.

Appendix 3
REFERENCES, USEFUL RESOURCES AND FURTHER READING

REFERENCES

BBC Health (2011) 'Depression in children.' London: BBC Health. Available at www.bbc.co.uk/health/emotional_health/mental_health/disorders_depression_child2.shtml, accessed on 13 September 2011.

Bowlby, J. (1969) *Attachment and Loss. Volume 1.* London: Hogarth Press.

Chazan, S. (2002) *Profiles of Play: Assessing and Observing Structure and Process in Play Therapy.* London: Jessica Kingsley *Publishers.*

Erikson, E.H. (1959) *Identity and the Life Cycle.* Psychological Issues Monograph. New York: International Universities Press.

Jennings, S. (1994) 'Models of practice in dramatherapy.' *British Association of Dramatherapists Journal of Dramatherapy 7,* 1, 1–5.

Jennings, S. (1999) *Introduction to Developmental Playtherapy: Playing and Health.* London: Jessica Kingsley *Publishers.*

Kellerman, P.F. and Hudgins, M.K. (2000) *Psychodrama with Trauma Survivors: Acting Out Your Pain.* London: Jessica Kingsley *Publishers.*

Lahad, M. (1992) 'Story-making in assessment method for coping with stress: six-piece story making and BASIC Ph.' In S. Jennings (ed.) *Dramatherapy Theory and Practice 2.* London: Routledge.

Lahad, M. (2000) *Creative Supervision. The Use of Expressive Arts Methods in Supervision and Self-Supervision.* London: Jessica Kingsley *Publishers.*

Landy, R. (1993) *Persona and Performance. The Meaning of Role in Dramatherapy and Everyday Life.* London: Jessica Kingsley *Publishers.*

Levine, P. (1997) *Waking the Tiger: Healing Trauma.* Berkeley, CA: North Atlantic Books.

LGfL (The Lancashire Grid for Learning) (2011) 'SEAL – Social and emotional aspects of learning.' Available at www.lancsngfl.ac.uk/nationalstrategy/ks3/behaveattend/index.php?category_id=37&s=!B121cf29d70ec8a3d54a33343010cc2, accessed on 12 October 2011.

McFarlane, P. (2005) *Dramatherapy: Developing Emotional Stability.* London: David Fulton Publishers Ltd.

McFarlane, P. and Harvey, J. (2012) *Dramatherapy and Family Therapy in Education: Essential Pieces of the Multi-Agency Jigsaw.* London: Jessica Kingsley *Publishers.*

NSPCC (National Society for the Prevention of Cruelty to Children) (2012) 'Domestic violence.' Available at www.nspcc.org.uk/inform/research/statistics/domesticabusewda87794html, accessed on 9 March 2012.

NSPCC (2011a) 'Prevalence and incidence of child abuse and neglect: Key child protection statistics.' Available at www.nspcc.org.uk/Inform/research/statistics/prevalence_and_incidence_of_child_abuse_and_neglect_wda48740.html, accessed on 23 September 2011.

NSPCC (2011b) 'Definition of child neglect.' Available at www.nspcc.org.uk/inform/resourcesforprofessionals/neglect_defintion_wda80232.html, accessed on 23 November 2011.

Piaget, J. (1970) 'Piaget's theory.' In P.H. Mussen (ed.) *Carmichael's Manual of Child Psychology, Volume 1.* New York: John Wiley Publishers.

Separation Statistics (2009) 'Separated families matter.' Available at www.separatedfamiliesmatter.org.uk/why-work-with-separation/separation-research, accessed on 23 November 2011.

Sunderland, M. (2006) *The Science of Parenting.* London: Jessica Kingsley *Publishers.*

USEFUL RESOURCES

Anxiety: www.youngminds.org.uk

Attachment: Pearce, C. (2009) *A Short Introduction to Attachment and Attachment Disorder.* London: Jessica Kingsley *Publishers.*

Autism: Taylor, P. (2011) *A Beginner's Guide to Autism Spectrum Disorders.* London: Jessica Kingsley *Publishers.*

Bullying: www.kidscape.org.uk; www.kidpower.org; www.kidshealth.org (dealing with bullies). See also Rigby, K. (2002*) Stop the Bullying.* London: Jessica Kingsley *Publishers.*

Depression: www.youngminds.org.uk

Nightmares: see www.dreamcatchers.org

Parental separation: www.changingfamilies.org.uk

Speech problems: www.ace-centre.org.uk; www.kidshealth.org

Trauma and shock: for effects of television see www.med.umich/yourchild/topics/tv.htm

FURTHER READING

Day, J. (1994) *Creative Visualization with Children: A Practical Guide.* Shaftesbury: Element Books.

Gerhardt, S. (2004) *Why Love Matters: How Affection Shapes a Baby's Brain.* Hove: Brunner-Routledge.

Jennings, S. (1986) *Creative Drama in Groupwork.* Bicester: Winslow Press.

Thomas, B. (2009) *Creative Coping Skills for Children: Emotional Support through Arts and Crafts Activities.* London: Jessica Kingsley *Publishers.*

INDEX

1, 2, 3 exercise 64–5

abandonment 69, 123
abstract concepts, difficulties
    with 31, 32, 69, 88
abuse 42–8
    activities 45–8
    behaviours 43–5
    domestic 23, 31, 98, 103
    issues 23, 34, 42–3
    quantifying 107
acceptance, as a stage of grief
    68
acknowledgement activities,
    for groups 144–5
adrenaline rushes 140
Adverb Game 149
age, chronological 29
age-related behaviour
    68–9, 93, 116–17, 123,
    124–5
aggression, as an area of
    concern 24, 45, 70, 77,
    108, 126, 141
aggressive behaviour 24, 48,
    97, 123, 129, 140
alcohol, addiction to 93
Alien Puppet exercise 131–2
alter ego, creating an 85
anger
    activities 48–9, 50–4
    behaviours 23, 49–50
    mirroring 140
    as a stage of grief 67–8
Angry Man exercise 50–1
anorexia 45
anxiety

activities 54–8, 56–8
    behaviours 23, 55–6, 140
    issues 54–5
anxiety disorders 56, 141
appetite, loss of 77
approval, over-dependence
    on 60
art activities 49, 74
art therapists 23, 33
arts projects 23
Asperger's syndrome 30, 123,
    129
assessment, suggestions for
    25–6
assimilation, as a stage of
    grief 68
attachment 58–65
    activities 60–5
    behaviours 59–60
    issues 23, 58–9
    mother and child 17–18
Attachment Theory 58
attention
    gaining 26, 88, 124
    seeking 65, 76, 108, 123
    sharing 27
Australia
    divorce statistics 115
    SEAL programme in 23
autism 30, 84, 123, 129
awareness exercises 132–3

Babes in the Wood exercise
    126–7
babyish behaviour 124
Back to Back exercise 62
BBC Health website 91

bed wetting 45, 55, 67, 76,
    93, 116, 141
beginning a session 39–41
Beginning, Middle and End
    exercise 120–1
behaviour, severe case
    scenarios 26–7
belief systems 104
Belly Breathing exercise 146
Ben's Bag of Worries exercise
    56–7
bereavement 66–74
    activities 71–4
    anxiety about 24, 30, 56
    behaviours 29, 66–70, 104
    issues 66
Best and Worst exercise 39
'big feelings' 49, 50, 55, 58,
    94, 112, 124
biological issues 91
blame
    attributing 70, 117, 125
    self-blame 30, 92, 116
body language
    and bullying 75, 77–9,
    82–3
    inappropriate 130
body sculpting 74, 121
bonding games 149–50
boredom 124
boundaries, setting
    behavioural 69, 116
Bowlby, John 58
brain
    benefits of physical exercise
    to 93

brain *cont.*
  chemicals 54, 55, 96, 98,
    123
  damage to 49, 59
  effect of trauma on 140–1
  hemispheres 35, 147
  higher 49, 55, 59, 141
  limbic 140
  lower 49, 55, 59, 97, 140
  making connections in 131
  processing issues 134
  stress hormones in 49, 59,
    112, 140
breathing exercises 48, 51,
  52–3, 54, 101, 143,
  145–8
Broken Record exercise 81,
  101–2
bulimia 45
bullying 75–83
  activities 77–83, 101–2
  behaviours 76–7, 129
  issues 23, 75–6, 92, 116,
    135

calming activities 27, 49,
  145–8
Candle Breathing exercise
  148
care, defining acceptable 107
carers, separation from 55
caring, compulsive 59
cathartic activities 49
CBT (cognitive behavioural
  therapy) 54
change 83–7
  activities 85–7
  behaviours 24, 85, 91
  issues 26, 29, 45, 56, 77,
    83–4, 92
Changing Families project
  115
Changing the Ending exercise
  113–14
Changing the Play exercise
  82–3, 121
Changing the Rhythm
  exercise 41
Chazan, Saralea 17
chemicals, in the brain 54,
  55, 96, 98, 123

child protection issues 42,
  89, 120
cities, inner-city arts project
  23
clay, working with 86, 95,
  128
clinging behaviour 59, 93,
  116
Close Eyes and Point exercise
  145
closure activities 143–5
coalition 123
coercion, in play 44, 141
cognitive behavioural therapy
  (CBT) 54
cohabitation 115
coldness, when angry 49–50
communication
  through metaphor 21,
    24, 32
  through play 17
  see also speech problems
compulsive caring 59
compulsive lying 32, 87–91
  activities 89–91
  behaviours 88–9
  issues 88
computer games, violence in
  31, 139
computer use 39, 134
confidence *see* lack of self-
  esteem/confidence;
  self-confidence
conflict resolution 126, 128
Consequences exercise 105–6
control issues 34, 46–7, 76,
  85
coping strategies 117
copying 28, 103, 129
  see also mirroring
cortisol 49, 59
Counting Up exercise 41
coverage, of book 20–2
craft activities 74, 128
Creative Expression Model 33
criticism, sensitivity to 88, 89
cruelty 97, 111
crying, as a sign of depression
  68, 93, 113
cultural awareness 29, 104,
  130

cyber bullying 75

danger, courting 93
death 69, 74, 91
  see also bereavement
demonization 125
denial
  being in 67, 73, 140
  denial skills 79
depression 91–6
  activities 94–6
  behaviours 92–3, 140
  issues 45, 76, 91–2, 107,
    118
deroling 35–6, 83, 100, 120,
  121, 122, 128
Desert Island exercise 127–8
developmental issues 29–30,
  108, 134
directive intervention 34
disbelief
  as a stage of grief 67
  suspension of 137
discipline, problems accepting
  103
displacement activities 25,
  28, 95
dissociation 141
Divided Room/Fibs and Fact
  exercise 89–90
Diving for Lands activity
  136–7
divorce
  statistics 115
  see also parental separation
doctors and nurses, playing
  44
domestic violence 23, 31,
  98, 103
doubling 36, 119, 121
Dragon Story 72–4
drama techniques, using 35–7
dramatic distancing 34, 35,
  119
dream catchers 114
dreams 32, 70
  see also nightmares
drug-taking 59, 93

eating issues 45, 93

embodiment, stage of development 33, 94–5
emotion, lack of 49–50, 59, 97–8
emotional abuse 42, 44
emotional development 137
emotional issues 39, 58, 134
emotional literacy, building 39
emotional support, drama techniques for 35–7
emotional trauma 29, 33
empathy
   encouraging 132–3
   lack of 97, 130
empowerment 114
ending a session 143–8
   calming activities 145–8
   closure activities 143–5
energy, releasing 52–4, 140, 145–6
Erikson, E.H. 33
Escape from a Prison of War Camp exercise 129
exclusions, from school 23
exercises see *titles of individual exercises*
expression, of anger 48
externalising
   anxieties 57, 58
   worries 57
extra-curricular activities 93, 118
eye contact 41, 64–5, 135

fact, and fantasy 31–2, 88–9
factual evidence 22
fairness 124
fairy stories 91, 109–10
Family Photo exercise 118–20
family reorganization 115–16, 118
fantasy, and fact 31–2, 88–9
favouritism 123, 125
fear, and nightmares 111
feel-good factor 55, 96, 98
feelings
   'big feelings' 49, 50, 55, 58, 112, 124

externalising 50–1, 57, 94–5
Fibs and Fact exercise 89–90
fight or flight 97, 140
fighting, among siblings 124, 125
films
   fantasy in 88
   horror 93
   violence in 31, 139
flashbacks 70, 141
freeze frames 36, 82, 102, 114, 119, 120, 121, 122
friendship issues 130
fright 59–60

genetic issues 55, 91, 134
Gorilla Breathing exercise 147–8
grief 66–74
   complicated 66, 70, 115–16
   echoing parents' 104
   simple 66–9
      age-related behaviour 68–9
      stages of 67–8
   see also bereavement
group acknowledgement activities 144–5
group bonding games 149–50
Group Fall exercise 63
group massage 144
Group Mime 149–50
group participation exercises 41
group sculpts 74
guessing games 25–6
guilt
   and depression 92
   and grief 67–8, 69

Harvey, J. 22
hatred 98
hearing loss 134
Helper exercise 109–10
hiding 60, 85
homelessness 92
horror, predilection for 93

hot seating 36, 119
Hudgins, M.K. 35
Hula Hoops game 40
hyperactivity 67, 140, 141
hyperventilation 145
hypervigilance 60, 140, 141

'I Need You to Listen' exercise 81
identity, issues 33, 48, 76, 96, 124
illness, as a factor in depression 91
illnesses, inventing 76, 84
'I'm OK' game 77–9
impulsive behaviour 123, 140
In the Mirror exercise 80
inhibition 44, 60, 96
insecure/ ambivalent attachments 59
insecure attachments 58, 59
insecure/ avoidant attachments 59
insecure/ disorganized attachments 59–60
insomnia 67
Institute of Dramatherapy 31
introductory exercises 39–40
irritability 68, 92, 93, 132
issues 23–37
   assessment suggestions 25–6
   a child's concept of reality 29–31
   drama techniques 35–7
   fact and fantasy 31–2
   general and differentiated approaches 28–9
   presenting behaviours 24
   research findings 23
   severe case scenarios 26–7
   underpinnings of dramatherapy 32–4
      directive and non-directive intervention 34
      dramatic distancing 34
      metaphor and symbol 32–3
      stages of development 33–4

Jailers exercise 64
Jennings, Sue 17–18, 33

Kellerman, P.F. 35

lack of self-esteem/
    confidence 96–102
    activities 99–102
    behaviours 97–8
    issues 96–7
Lahad, Mooli 31, 109
Lancashire Grid for Learning
    (LGfL) 23
Landy, R. 34
language development 135
learning difficulties, children
    with 131
learnt behaviour 103–6
    activities 105–6
    behaviours 104, 129
    issues 103–4
letters, writing to the
    deceased 74
Levine, Peter 96–7, 140
LGfL (Lancashire Grid for
    Learning) 23
life skills 126
loss 48
    see also bereavement
love, issues surrounding 32,
    96, 97–8, 111
lying 45
    see also compulsive lying

Magic Thumb exercise 25
manipulation issues 125
massage, group 144
materials 20
McFarlane, P. 22, 28
Me in my Bubble exercise
    132–3, 145
meditation 147
memory boxes 74
metaphor 24, 56, 57, 73,
    91, 95
metaphor and symbol 32–3
mime, for groups 149–50
mirroring 36, 80, 81,
    139–40
    see also copying
monsters 33, 88, 112, 114
    overcoming 46–7

moods, sensitivity to 92, 93
Motorway exercise 144
moving on, as a stage of
    grief 68
Mr. Angry Man exercise 50–1
mummies and daddies,
    playing 44
My Hero exercise 99–101
myths 93

nail biting 55
National Society for the
    Prevention of Cruelty to
    Children (NSPCC) 42,
    107, 108, 139
neglect 106–11
    activities 109–11
    behaviours 107–8
    in early childhood 96–7
    as a form of abuse 42
    issues 23, 106–7
negotiation skills 127–8
nervous habits 77
nervous system 55
neurological issues 134
neuroses 54, 55
night terrors 112
nightmares 45, 55, 56, 76,
    111–15, 141
    activities 113–15
    behaviours 112–13
    issues 111–12
non-directive intervention
    34, 73
normalization 60, 117, 118
NSPCC (National Society
    for the Prevention of
    Cruelty to Children) 42,
    107, 108, 139
numbness 67, 141

Office for National Statistics
    115
omission, bullying by 76
One, Two, Three, Four
    breathing exercise 147
online help 76
Opposite Corners exercise
    94–5
oproids 55, 96
over-protectiveness 44, 55

overbearing adult behaviour
    34
overdosing 93
oxytocin 55, 96

panic attacks 141
parental separation 115–22
    activities 118–22
    behaviours 115–18
    issues 23, 115
Parts of the Body game 150
persistence, in bullying 75–6
pervasive anxiety 55
phobias 54, 55, 57–8, 141
    school 24, 56, 76, 84, 92
physical abuse 42, 43
physical contact
    and building trust 61–5
    caution using 61, 144
physical exercise 40, 93, 118
physiological issues 134
Piaget, Jean 32, 33
Pinocchio 91
play therapists 33, 60
please, desire to 88, 89, 98,
    99
Pneumatic Drill game 40
polarization
    within a family 123, 125
    of views on sexes 104
pornography 43
potty training 93
poverty 92
power
    activities for re-establishing
    46–7
    of bullies 76
praise, problems with 96
presenting behaviours 24
projection, stage of
    development 33, 131,
    140
promiscuity 60
protection mechanisms 46–7,
    116
PSHE (Personal Social
    Health and Economic
    education) 75
psyches, children's 111
psychodrama 35

psychodynamic intervention 23
psychological development 29, 137
psychomatic symptoms 60, 140
psychoses 50, 54
psychotherapy 54
PTSD (post-traumatic stress disorder) 70, 139
punishment, sensitivity to 89
puppets 25, 28, 29, 33, 97, 110, 131–2
Push Hands exercise 63

quality of life 56

rapid eye movement (REM) sleep 112
re-traumatization 35, 114
readership, of the book 18–20
reality
    avoiding 89
    boundaries with fantasy 31–2
    a child's concept of 29–31
    transition between imaginative play and 39–40
reason, inability to 49
reframing 36, 79, 82–3, 91
Reframing/Trying Again exercise 121–2
regression 26–7
rejection 60, 65, 92, 123
relaxation 49, 54
REM (rapid eye movement) sleep 112
repetition
    as a cause for concern 26, 70, 135, 141
    as a means of support 85, 86
resentment 124–5
resilience, developing 99, 107, 109
resources, necessary 20
reunion, normalizing 60
ritualistic actions 39–40, 86–7, 143

rivalry see sibling rivalry
role, stage of development 33–4, 97
role models 103–4, 106
role reversal 37, 81
routine, benefits of 39
running 48

safe rooms 48–9
safeguarding 22, 89, 107
salt sculptures 74
Saucepan exercise 52–3, 145
'Say My Name Like...' exercise 145
scapegoating 44
school
    exclusions from 23
    phobia about 24, 56, 76, 84, 92
school issues 25–6, 75, 116, 123
sculpting 37, 74, 119, 121
sculptures 74, 86, 95, 128
SEAL (social and emotional aspects of learning) programme 23
seasons of nature 74
secrets 45
secure attachments 58–9
self-awareness 33, 33–4, 124
self-blame 92
self-confidence 92, 141
self-empowerment 99, 101
self-esteem 141
    building 46–7, 141
    see also lack of self-esteem/ confidence
self-exploration 33
self-harm 45, 77, 93
self-healing 73
self-reliance 60
self-worth 60, 76, 92
SEN (special educational needs), teachers 19
sensitivity, over-sensitivity 92
sensory motors 33
separation
    from carers 55
    insecure attachments 58
    and loss 67
    normalizing 60

parental
    and dramatic distancing 34, 35
    effect on children 29–30, 30, 56, 84, 91
    issue in inner-city arts project 23
    and loss 66
    of self from others 30, 33–4
Separation Statistics 115
sessions, beginning see beginning a session
severe behavioural case scenarios 26–7
sexes, polarization of views on 104
sexual abuse 43, 44–5
sexual behaviour, premature 103, 129
sexuality, teenagers and 116–17
Shield activity 46–7, 87
shock
    as a stage of grief 67
    trauma of 97
shyness 96
sibling rivalry 122–9
    activities 126–9
    behaviours 124–6
    issues 122–4
sick, fear of being 57–8
singing 86, 136, 138
sleep 76, 112
social and emotional aspects of learning (SEAL) programme 23
social cues 130–1
socially inappropriate behaviour 129–34
    activities 131–4, 136–8
    behaviours 130–1, 135–6
    issues 129–30, 134
space
    awareness of 132–3
    inappropriate use of 130
    requirements 19–20
speaking from role 37, 83
special educational needs see SEN

special schools 26
'special' time 126
speech and language
    therapists 134
speech problems 134–8
splitting 85, 140
stammering 77, 135
Status Game/I'm OK 77–9
stealing 77, 92, 108
stepfamilies 117, 125
storymaking 28, 72–4, 87,
    102, 109–10, 126–7
stress 23, 55, 92, 113
stress hormones 49, 59, 112,
    140
stuttering 77, 135
suicide 45, 76, 77, 104
Sunderland, Margot 49, 55,
    96, 123
supervision guidelines 108
swearing 129
sweating 50
Sword in the Stone story 87
symbol and metaphor 32–3
symbolism 24, 29, 93, 95

Talking in Numbers exercise
    137–8
Tangles exercise 144–5
teasing 44, 135
television use 39, 134
therapists see *individual types
    of therapist*
threatened, feeling 123
Through the Wall story 28
thumping cushions 48
tics 77
training required 19
transference 125
transition
    between reality and
        imaginative play
        39–40
    see also change or transition
trauma
    anxiety about 24
    in early childhood 96–7
    emotional 29, 33
    as a factor in depression 91
    using psychodrama to
        treat 35

trauma and shock 139–41
    behaviours 139–41
    issues 139
triggers 27, 56
truant, playing 92
trust
    building 27, 47, 60
    exercises 61–5, 141
    importance of 19
    mutual 144
trust versus mistrust 33
Truth game 25–6
Trying Again exercise 121–2
Two Islands exercise 85–6,
    87

Ugly Ducking storywork 102
UK (United Kingdom)
    divorce statistics 115
    SEAL programme in 23
unpredictability 59
unresponsiveness 93
USA (United States of
    America)
    divorce statistics 115
    SEAL programme in 23

violence
    as a consequence 59, 124
    and depression 92
    domestic
        effects of witnessing 31,
            103, 139–40
        issues 23
        unsuitable exercises 89
    effects of witnessing 31,
        139
    as socially inappropriate
        behaviour 129
    see also anger
visualizations 49, 54, 143,
    148
Volcano exercise 51–2 ·

warming up activities 40
weight change 93
Winnie the Pooh storywork
    102
Woodchopper breathing
    exercise 145–6
world

awareness of the outside
    33
ideal 88
taking time to enter the
    child's 28
yoga 147
You May Think this is a Piece
    of Material... exercise
    71–2

ACTING ON IMPULSE

Andrew Trim

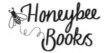

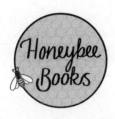

Published by Honeybee Books
www.honeybeebooks.co.uk

Printed in the UK using paper from sustainable sources

ISBN: 978-1-913675-38-7

Cover illustration by Sam Zambelli

@thatsrichartwork